Chu Gar Mantis

Lao Sui's Martial Art Legacy in China

劉水功夫遺產在中國

Southern Praying Mantis Kungfu

East River Chu Gar Mantis Clans
Lao Sui's Family and Pupils at
Lao's Huiyang, Guangdong Home, 2012

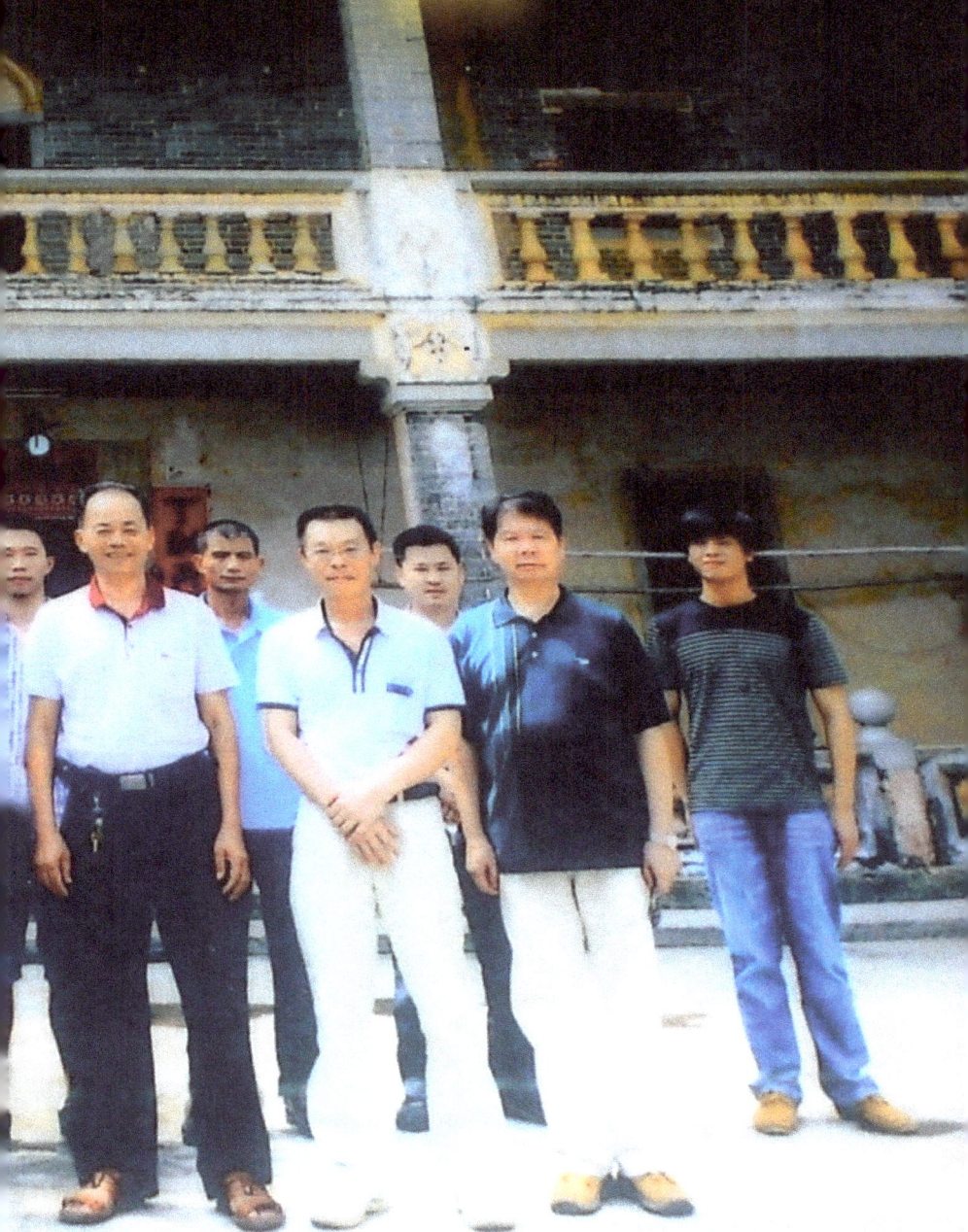

東江朱家螳螂清溪。盧州羅門
人於劉水宗師故居合照留念
2012

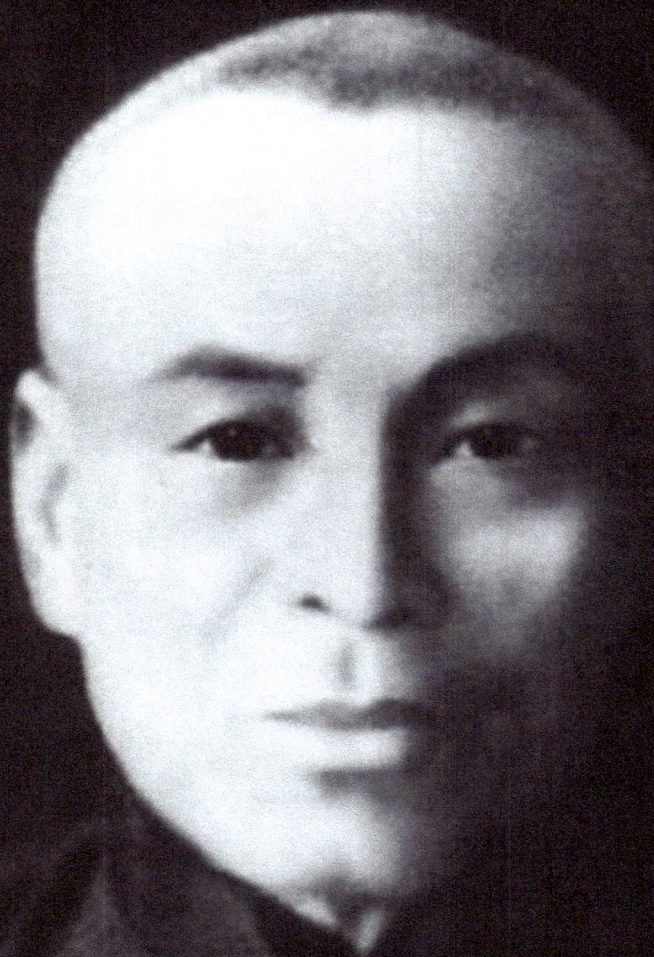

劉水師公遺像

Lao Sui

第三代傳人劉水

3rd Generation Chu Gar Gao
(1879 - 1942)

派螳蟷家朱

劉水功夫遺產在中國

Chu Gar Mantis

Lao Sui's Martial Art Legacy in China

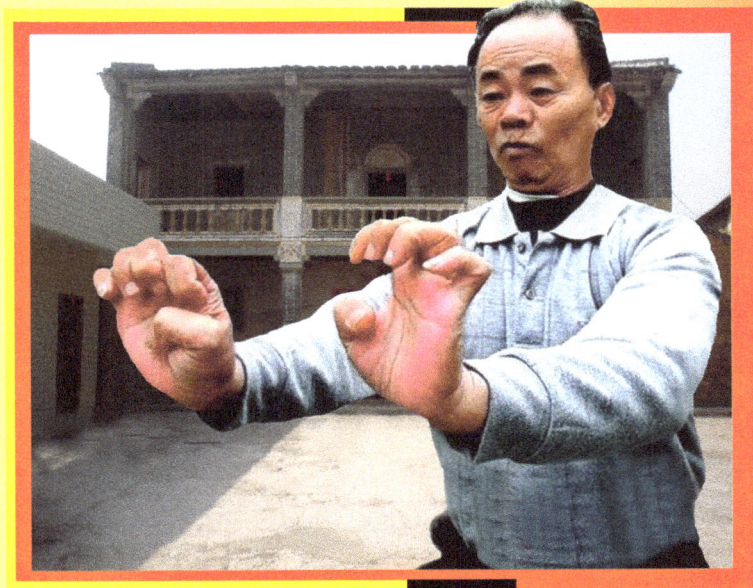

Featuring

Sifu Ma Jiu Hua　馬九華 師傅
Sifu Chen Jian Ming　陳建明 師傅
Sifu Xie Tian Sheng　謝添勝 師傅

By
Roger D. Hagood

Charles Alan Clemens, Sean Robinson, Editors

Southern Mantis Press ┃ Pingshan Town, China

著作版權所有 **Copyright © 2013 by Roger D. Hagood**

Southern Mantis Press
462 W. Virginia St. (Rt. 14)
Crystal Lake, Illinois 60014
1-800-Jook Lum
books@southernmantispress.com

Ordering Information:
Special discounts are available for martial art schools, bookstores, specialty shops, museums and events. Contact the publisher at the email address above.

Cover photograph: Ma Jiuhua Sifu's late father, Ma Mingsen, was married to Lao Sui's daughter. Ma Sifu's family are still next door neighbors to the Lao family and remain in the old Lao Sui village today.

封面照片：馬九華師傅
馬九華師傅的父親馬銘森娶劉水的女兒為妻，至今在香園村馬師傅仍與劉水後人比鄰而居。

ISBN: 978-0-9857240-6-1
Chu Gar Mantis: Lao Sui's Martial Art Legacy in China

Dedication 獻言

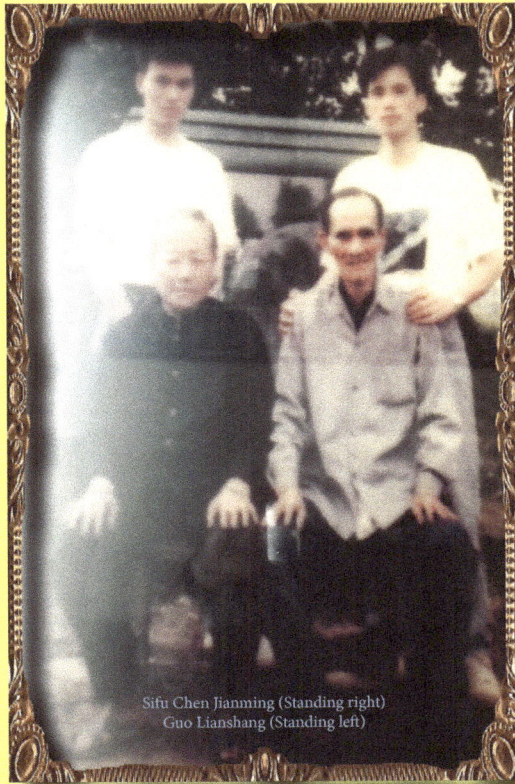

Sifu Chen Jianming (Standing right)
Guo Lianshang (Standing left)

Late Chu Gar Master Ma Mingsen and wife seated
Huiyang, Huizhou, China
Son-in-law of Lao Sui

Late Ma Mingsen Sifu

The very hometown where Lao Sui's Chu Gar came from would likely be without Chu Gar today, if Ma Mingsen had not returned in 1941 and eventually taught the Art to his fellow villagers. After 30 years of complete secrecy, he finally opened up and imparted Chu Gar to others in the place from whence it came. The Lao and Ma families were always related by location and marriage. Ma Sifu was married to Lao Sui's daughter! Today the descendants of Lao Sui and Ma Mingsen carry on Chu Gar in their hometown of Huiyang, Huizhou, China under Ma's family and disciples.

獻言 – 馬銘森 師傅
朱家螳螂拳故馬銘森師傅留影於劉水宗師的故鄉–中國廣東省惠州市惠陽區

如果沒有馬銘森師傅，朱家螳螂拳在劉水宗師的故鄉可能已經失傳，懷抱著使命感和寬廣的胸襟回到惠陽縣，馬銘森師傅將劉水宗師密傳的朱家螳螂拳廣泛地傳播於廣東省惠陽縣，身為劉水宗師的傳人與東床至親，兼桃兩家傳承，至今其後人仍於劉水宗師的故鄉中國廣東省惠州市惠陽區致力於朱家螳螂拳的傳遞。

Dedication 奉獻

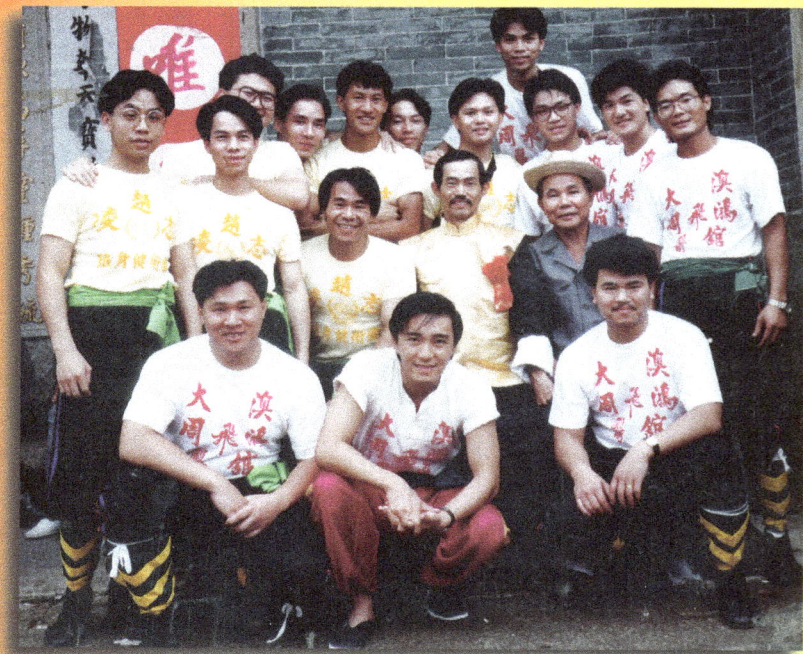

Late Sifu Cheng Wan

As Ma Mingsen was responsible for keeping Chu Gar alive in Lao Sui's home village, so was Cheng Wan chiefly responsible for Chu Gar in Hong Kong after Chu Kwong Hua's passing. Cheng Sifu tirelessly promoted Chu Gar Mantis in the press, events, and television. Notice Cheng Sifu in the hat above on set with "Kungfu Hustle" movie star Stephen Chau (Zhou Xing-Chi) (front and center kneeling). And that is Cheng Chiu, Sifu's son, standing to his left.

Every year for 35 years, in the summer, Cheng Sifu held Chu Gar Mantis celebrations with hundreds of international kungfu teachers, students, laymen, and laywomen in attendance. They were grand traditional kungfu celebrations of the old type.

Cheng Sifu also was from Lao Sui's home area in Huiyang and he often travelled back to Huiyang and visited with Ma Jiuhua Sifu and the others there. And Ma Sifu and brothers from Huiyang also visited Cheng Sifu in Hong Kong. A brother-friendship existed among the Hong Kong and Huiyang Chu Gar clans and everyone recognized each other as one family of Lao Sui's martial art legacy.

Cheng Sifu was old fashioned and yet high-tech. He was Hakka with international friends. And - he was my Sifu by ceremony. Fewer and fewer are the masters of the old tradition today, even here, in Hong Kong and China. –RDH

故鄭運師傅

一如馬銘森師傅延續劉水宗師在廣東的傳承，朱冠華師傅邊歸道山後，鄭運師傅是香港朱家螳螂拳承先啟後的關鍵人物，鄭運師傅不辭艱辛透過多種媒體推廣朱家螳螂拳，（照片帶帽者即為鄭運師傅，右坐蓄鬍者即元華，前排中跪立者即"功夫"男主角周星馳，鄭運師傅的兒子則立於他左邊，過去三十五年每年的夏天，鄭運師傅都會主辦朱家螳螂拳年會，來自於世界各國數百名功夫教師，學生 及初入門者躬逢盛會。

鄭運師傅的故鄉也在惠陽區，他經常回到惠陽，並拜會馬九華師傅和其他同門，馬九華師傅也常偕同門到香港與鄭運師傅交流。經由劉水宗師的傳承，香港和惠陽朱家螳螂拳門人同氣連枝。

鄭師傅是念舊但心胸開闊不守舊的現代科技人，他是客家人但擁有許多國際友人，我有幸忝列門牆之下，親受其熏炙，隨著他乘鶴西歸後，我越來越難遇到像他一樣的典範。 -RDH

kwongsaimantis.com

Contents

本書內容

Southern Mantis Ancestral Shrine

Chu Gar Praying Mantis Kungfu Creed

Hoc Yurn; Hoc Yi; Hoc Kungfu

學仁　學義　學功夫

Jurn Jow; Jurn Si; Jurn Gow Do

尊親　尊師　尊教訓

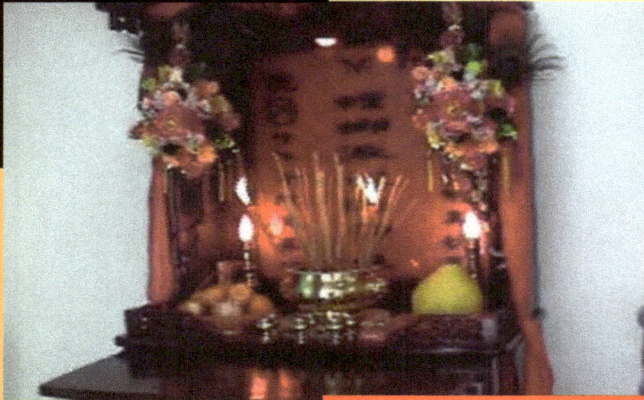

Respect the Ancestors for their transmission of the art.
尊敬歷代祖師 － 武術的傳承。

Respect the Sifu for his teaching.
尊敬師傅 － 他的教學。

Respect the Older Brothers for their dedication and loyalty.
尊敬同門師兄 － 他們的奉獻和忠誠。

Respect the Younger Brothers for determination in training.
尊敬同門師弟 － 他們堅毅的決心

Preface

This book is the culmination of some 36 years of personal effort in Southern Praying Mantis and 46 years of martial arts training and teaching. For those with the slightest interest in Southern Praying Mantis Kungfu, the name of Lao Sui holds the mystique of an old fashioned kungfu master who was revered by all to the extent he is often referred to as a "Canton Tiger." Lao Sui's legacy in China has always been called Chu Gar Mantis, just as it is today!

This book is published to unite and not to divide his teaching. It is to illuminate and not to hold in secret. It is to reveal the fact from the fiction about Lao Sui's legacy of martial art in China.

And we should remember there are other brother-friends in Chu Gar Mantis which are not descended from ancestor Lao Sui's teaching, but from a separate stream of Wong Fook Go's teaching.

Whatever you call Lao Sui's legacy today, Chu, Chow, or East River Hakka Mantis, it all comes from one place and one person - Lao Sui. In China, Lao's family, pupils, and villagers have always called his legacy Chu Gar Mantis. Let brother-friendship and harmony be the rule and everyone recognize Lao Sui's teaching as one family and Pai.

RDH
Guangdong, China
Spring, 2013

前言

這本書是累積個人近四十年的努力和研究的最終成果，對南螳螂拳稍有涉獵的人都聽過劉水的名字 – 神祕的傳統功夫大師，他的功夫受到極度的推崇，被尊稱為廣東之虎。

這本書的出版是為了對劉水畢生教學做一整合而非製造分歧，是發揚分享而非閉門自珍。由流傳的支字片語中一窺劉水 宗師的全貌，我們也應該記得朱家螳螂拳除劉水 宗師一脈之外，還有許多黃福高祖師再傳的同門兄弟。

今天無論你怎麼稱呼劉水 宗師留給後人的遺產，朱家，周家或東江客家螳螂拳，所有一切都來自於同一個地方 – 廣東省惠陽縣！讓我們遵循同門情誼與和諧的原則，所有傳承自劉水 宗師的人皆份屬同門。

RDH, 中國廣東省， 2013年春

從何處來：地理位置

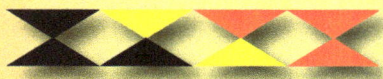

From Whence We Came: Location

劉水和客家螳螂拳發源地的地理位置

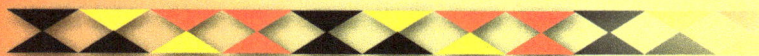

土地富饒民風淳樸的發源地

客家拳是指傳承於中國南方省份(包括廣東省-地圖中紅標處)的客家族群中的傳統武術, 大致包括：Liujiaquan(劉家拳), Diaojiaquan(刁家拳), Zhongjiaquan(鐘家拳), Lijiaquan(李家拳), Yuejiaquan(岳家拳), Liuminquan(流民拳), Liu Fengshan Pai(劉鳳山派), Kunlunquan(崑崙拳), Niujiaquan (牛家拳), 各門派使用的武器則有：gun(槍), gan(桿), shungdao(雙刀), tiechi(鐵尺), gou(勾)lian(鐮), katou(卡頭)和dado(大刀)。

Zhujiaquan(朱家拳), Kwongsai Jook Temple(江西竹林寺)和Iron Ox(鐵牛)三派客家拳常被統稱為南螳螂拳, 這三派南螳螂拳不僅有著相似的術語命名, 也依循共通的武術原則, 基礎, 和技擊慣例。

Chu Gar Mantis Cities in Southern China
Guangdong, Province

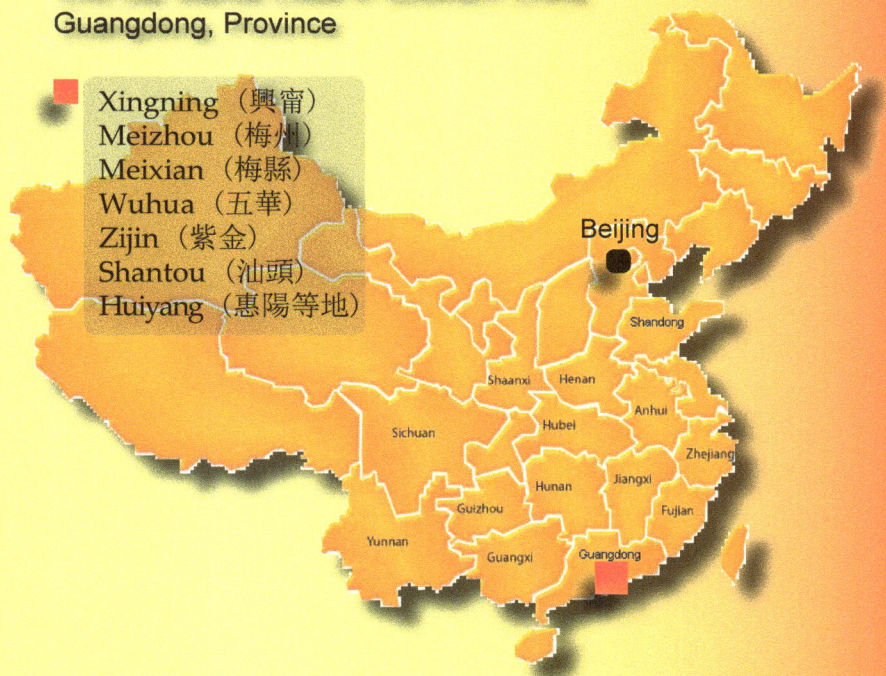

Xingning （興寗）
Meizhou （梅州）
Meixian （梅縣）
Wuhua （五華）
Zijin （紫金）
Shantou （汕頭）
Huiyang （惠陽等地）

Beijing

Shandong

Shaanxi   Henan

Sichuan   Hubei   Anhui

Zhejiang

Hunan   Jiangxi

Guizhou   Fujian

Yunnan   Guangxi   Guangdong

Lao Sui & Hakka Mantis on the Map

A Region of Kindness, Benefits, and Boxing

Kejiaquan (客家拳) or Hakka boxing, refers to a number of kungfu styles practiced by the ethnic Hakka people in China's Southern Provinces including Guangdong (red square above). Some of the Hakka styles include: Liujiaquan (刘家拳); Diaojiaquan (刁家拳); Zhongjiaquan (钟家拳); Lijiaquan (李家拳); Yuejiaquan (岳家拳); Liuminquan (流民拳); Liu Fengshan Pai (刘凤山派); Kunlunquan (昆仑拳); and Niujiaquan (牛家拳). Commonly used martial art weapons in Hakka styles are: gun (棍); gan (杆); shuangdao (双刀); tiechi (铁尺); gou (勾); lian (镰); Katou (卡 头) ; and the Dadao (大刀).

Zhujiaquan (朱家拳) Chu Gar; Kwongsai Jook Lum Temple (江

另一個共通性是它們的起源和傳承的地理位置, 客家螳螂所有三派彼此可謂近在咫尺, 都在今日的惠州市惠陽區。

廣東省惠州市(惠風和暢)

惠州市位於廣東省省會廣州市之東, 為粵東的主要城市之一, 明朝(公元1368年－1644年)時即稱惠州, 但自1958年起始升級為惠州市。

中國人常說地靈人傑, 惠州素以其地貌聞名於世包括綠山、 湖泊、 河流、 溫泉和瀑布, 以及許多廣為人知的歷史名人,

惠州是一個輸入埠和及東江流域的工業中心。 主要產業包括電子、 紡織、 醫藥、 煉糖、 食品加工、 飲料、 塑膠和精密機械。中國最大的外資之一碰巧也是位於廣東省惠州市的美國石化公司。

國家公路和鐵路連接惠州市輿其其周圍的城市。 東江提供良好的內河運輸, 惠州市與香港相隔也只是幾個小時的路程。

惠州也以農業著稱, 盛產許多特有的蔬菜、酒、 家禽、 水果和海鮮。 遊客可以在此古老的城市盡情享受, 惠州也是許多客家武術的發源地。

而這恰好是朱家螳螂拳蓬勃發展和劉水武術遺產傳承之所在！

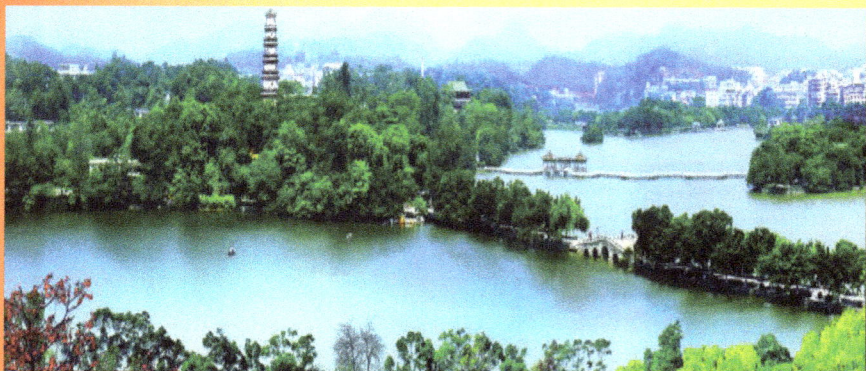

西竹林寺); and Iron Ox (鐵牛) are three types of Hakka Kungfu commonly called "Southern Praying Mantis (南螳螂)." These three styles of Southern Mantis boxing not only share similar nomenclature, but also have common principles, fundamentals, and boxing routines.

Another commonality is their location of origin and propagation. All three branches of Hakka Mantis are in close proximity to each other and Chu Gar Mantis, as we know it today, was fomented in Huizhou City, Huiyang District.

惠州 Huizhou (Favoured with Kindness and Benefit) Guangdong Province

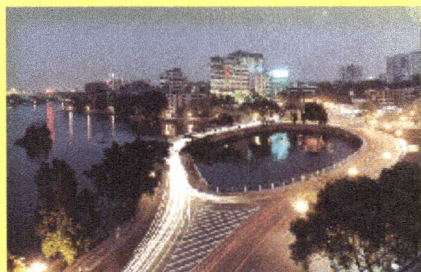

Huizhou is one of the major cities to the east of Guangzhou, the capital of Guangdong Province. It has been called Huizhou since the Ming Dynasty (1368 - 1644 AD), and recognized as a city in 1958.

As a Chinese saying goes: "Fertile land fosters talents". Huizhou is popular for its historic figures and celebrities as well as its landforms, which include green mountains, lakes, rivers, springs and waterfalls.

Huizhou is an entry port, as well as, an industrial center in the East River Valley. Electronics, textiles, medicine, sugar refining, food processing, beverages, plastics and precision machinery are among its light industries. China's largest foreign investment also happens to be in Huizhou, a USA petrochemical company.

National highways and railways connect Huizhou with its surrounding cities. The Dongjiang East River is good for navigation and Huizhou City is only a few hours from Hong Kong by air conditioned bus.

Agriculture is excellent and there are many Huizhou specialties of vegetables, wines, chickens, fruits, and seafood. It is one of the ancient cities in South China where visitors can enjoy themselves for

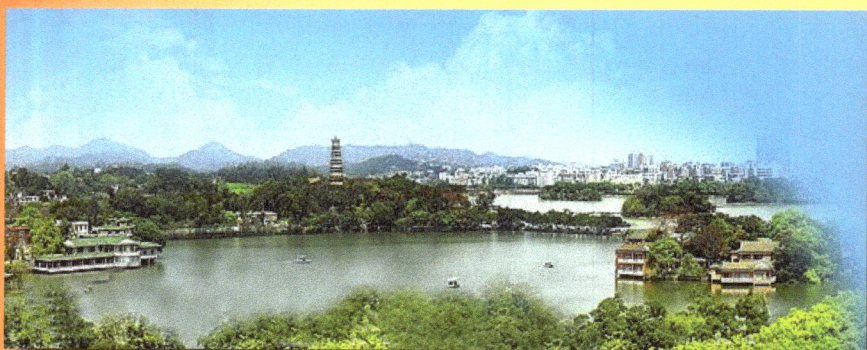

觀音閣-觀音寺

與惠陽劉水故居隔東江相望就是位於博羅縣的觀音寺, 博羅縣自古以來即名列廣東省四大縣之一。

大約公元1899年在觀音寺，二十歲的劉水遇見改變他一生的人-黃福高。

觀音閣是惠州市博羅縣縣府所轄十七個鎮之一。

鎮辦公室對面，位於東江邊即是觀音寺的入口。

每日均有許多遊客慕觀音寺之名前往觀音閣，但幾乎無人記得朱家螳螂拳的歷史 ！

觀音寺附近至今尚無告示牌簡介這段歷史。

今天的寺廟不同於劉水當年(公元1899年到1904年)在此地居住時的外貌，

原寺廟在文革期間被夷為平地，在九十年代初期在原址重建今日的寺廟。

山河依舊, 人事已非, 今日只有這滾滾東江和觀音閣見證朱家螳螂拳這段歷史。

days on end and definitely worth a visit, as it is also home to many Hakka boxing styles.

And it happens to be the location where Chu Gar Mantis blossomed and has become known worldwide as the martial art legacy of Lao Sui!

觀音閣 Guan Yin Ge - Temple of the Goddess of Mercy

Just across the East River from Lao Sui's home village in Huiyang is the Goddess of Mercy Temple in Boluo County. Boluo is recognized as one of four major ancient counties in Guangdong Province.

It was at this Guanyin Temple circa 1899, that Lao Sui as a young man of 20 met his Master, Wong Fook Go.

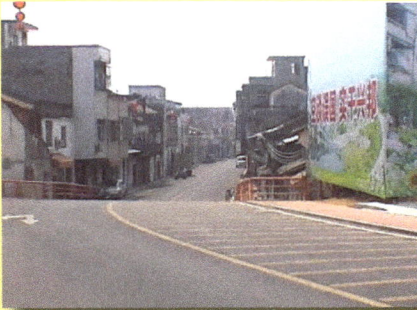
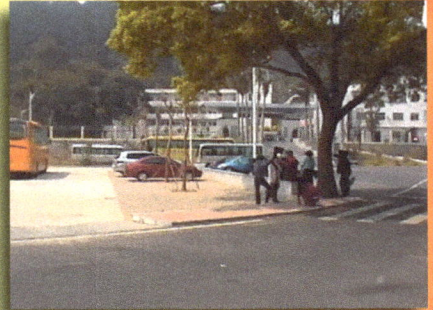

Above: Guanyin Temple Town is one of seventeen Towns which are administered by Boluo County government, Huizhou.

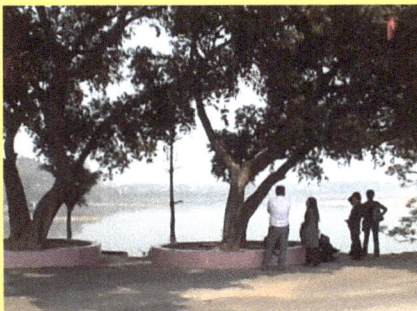
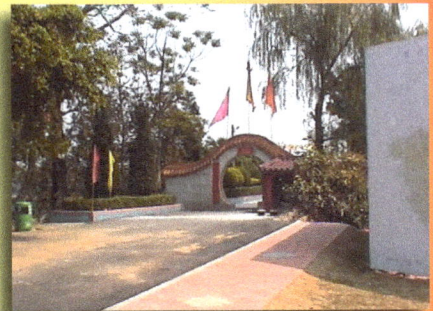

Above: Just opposite of the government office and situated on the East River is the entrance to the Temple.

19

觀音閣 Guan Yin Ge - Temple of the Goddess of Mercy

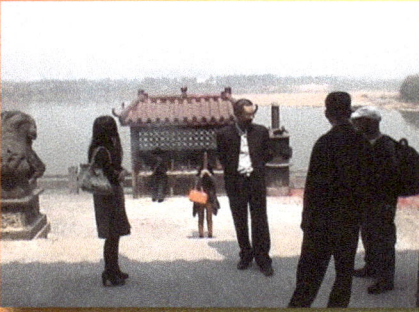

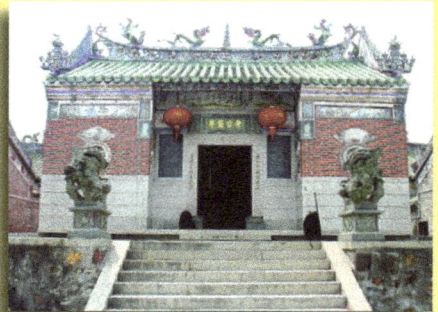

Above: Visitors are attracted to this Temple by tourist bus from nearby areas, largely unaware of it's past Chu Gar Mantis connection! There are no open signs or records of Chu Gar's transmission here.

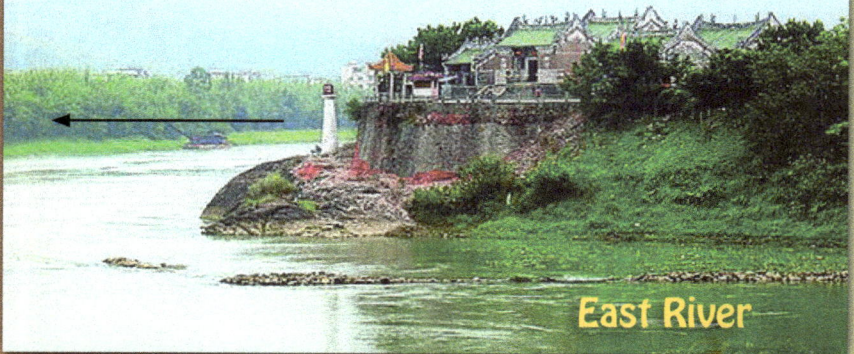

Just across the East River in the direction of the arrow is Lao Sui's old family home

East River

Above: The Temple today is dissimilar from Lao Sui's Chu Gar training days circa 1899-1904. During the cultural revolution the Temple was razed and then remodelled again in the early 1990s.

Today, the Temple of Goddess Guan Yin is related to Chu Gar Mantis only by virtue of its history of being the location where a young martial artist, Lao Sui, by chance, is said to have found the kungfu style called Chu Gar Gao under a small pier bridge on the East River.

20

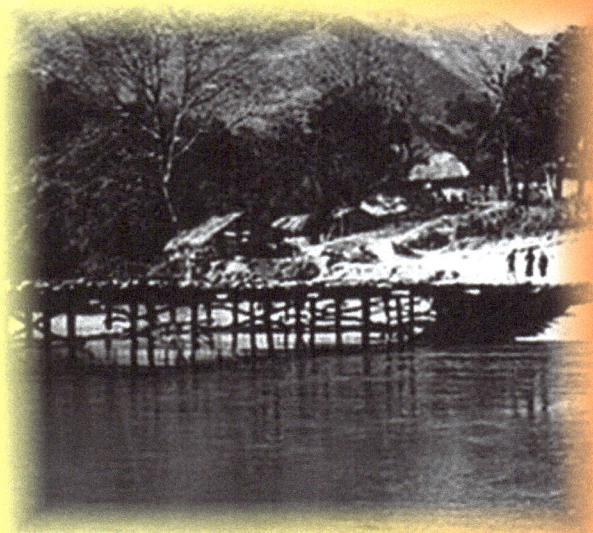

A Wandering Medicine Man

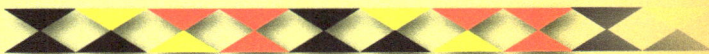

Lao Sui Finds Chu Gar Mantis Under A Bridge

The Chu Gar Mantis ancestor we commonly refer to as Lao Sui, has many names by which he may be referred to in Chinese. For clarification in this book, we will refer to him simply as Lao Sui.

Lao Sui was born in 1879, in Hong Yuen Village, Huiyang District, Huizhou City in China's southern Province of Guangdong. His hobby since childhood was martial arts and by the age of 20 he had gained quite a reputation. Particularly fond of staff play, his "Lao Sui Cudgel" was well known in the village.

Just across the East River, the people of Lao Sui's village often boated the short distance to Guan Yin Temple to attend village fairs and festivals. It is said that Lao Sui was always going to and fro at those times looking for boxing contests to join!

21

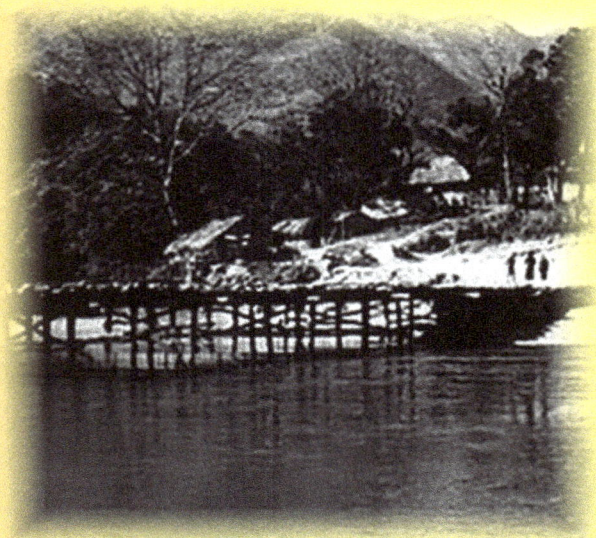

神奇的醫者

劉水在觀音閣橋下的巧遇

劉水一生致力推廣朱家螳螂拳, 使得朱家螳螂拳不再是局促一隅的地方武術, 一舉名列廣東十三名拳之一, 因此本門中人均奉劉水為祖師, 由於語言隔閡和傳統中國習俗(以字行), 在口語及文獻中他有許多不同的名字, 為避免混淆, 在這本書中一律稱他為劉水。

劉水於公元1879年出生於中國南方廣東省惠陽縣香園村, 他自小愛好武術, 在二十歲時他在地方上已小有名氣, 其中又以棍法著稱。

每逢觀音閣市集或是廟會時, 劉水故鄉的人均會乘船渡江參與盛會, 年輕的劉水也不例外常出現於這些場合, 四處尋找外來的武術家較技印證所學。

On one such occasion, Lao happened upon a wandering medicine seller under the pier bridge at Guan Yin Temple. The medicine man was named Wong Fook Go and he was a second generation master of Chu Gar Gao or Chu Family Creed boxing.

Wong was a wandering medicine seller from nearby Xingning City, who just happened to be journeying near Lao's home on a day when the young Lao was out and about looking for a boxing match.

Having heard Wong, the medicine seller, was good at kungfu, the young and fit Lao Sui engaged in a few rounds of boxing with Wong and was squarely defeated each time. Lao immediately bowed down to Wong Fook Go and requested to become his student. He was only 20 years old and the year is said to have been 1899.

For the next four years, under the careful guidance of Wong Fook Go, Lao Sui trained to be a perfect Southern Mantis boxer and also learned the use of guns, knives, and bone-setting medicine and so became known as the third-generation descendant of Chu Gar Southern Mantis.

In 1903, after four years of training with his Master at the Guan Yin Pavilion, the 24 year old Lao left his home in Huiyang and moved to Hong Kong where he worked for some 15 years before considering to teach Chu Gar.

By all accounts, it was circa 1918, when Lao Sui opened his first Chu Gar Mantis school in Hong Kong. For more information about Lao Sui's Hong Kong years, read my first book on Chu Gar Gao.

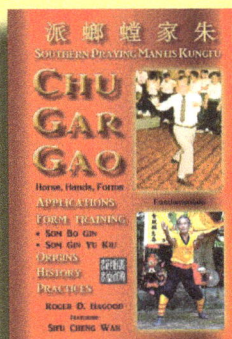

有一次劉水在觀音閣橋墩下遇到一位游走四方的醫者，他名叫黃福高是朱家螳螂拳第二代的傳人。

黃福高來自於粵北興甯市, 碰巧當天來到觀音閣, 遇到年輕熱衷於比試的劉水, 聽到黃福高也擅長功夫, 劉水不由技癢主動要求與黃福高試手, 但幾個回合比試劉水均敗北, 劉水立即向黃福高跪下懇求成為他的學生, 當時他年僅二十歲(公元1899 年)。

歷經四年, 在黃福高悉心指導下, 將劉水鍛鍊成精通南方螳螂拳的武術家, 同時也學會刀, 槍 和中醫傷科, 並成為朱家螳螂拳第三代傳人。

在1903年時二十四歲的劉水離開惠陽縣家鄉移居香港, 直到十五年後他才在香港公開傳授朱家螳螂拳。

大約是1918 年, 劉水在香港正式開設他的朱家螳螂拳學校。

有關劉水在香港的詳細資訊, 可閱讀我朱家螳螂拳的第一本書。

CHU GAR GAO 可於 AMAZON, BARNES & NOBLE, BOOK-A-MILLION 或其他大型書店郵購, 請以 "SOUTHERN MANTIS PRESS"關鍵詞搜尋。

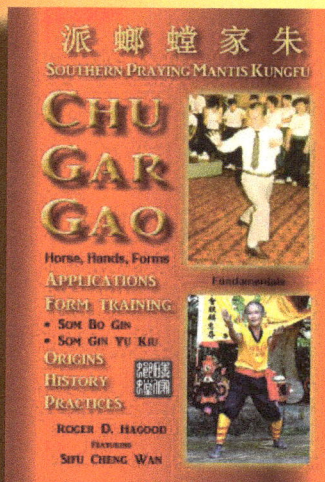

Briefly, it can be said that once Lao Sui opened his door to teach in Hong Kong, he had several groups of close students and hundreds of outer gate students and grand students.

Among those close to him were his son, Lao Wei Keung, Lao's Son-in-law, Ma Ming Sen, and others to include Yang Sao, Wu Yuan, Yip Hay, Chu Gwei, Chu Kwong Hua, Lam Hua, Tam Hua, Tam Chui, Sun Hsing, and Yip Sui. It was the late Sifu Yip Sui who carried forward Lao Sui's tradition under the name which has become known as Chow Gar. Lao Sui called his martial art Chu Gar Mantis and those in his hometown of Huiyang today (2013) still refer to the art as Chu Gar Mantis.

At age 30, Ma Ming Sen, who was married to Lao Sui's daughter in the village, travelled from Huiyang to Hong Kong by boat, down the East River. From 1937-1941, Ma stayed with Lao Sui in Hong Kong and concentrated on training the Chu Gar Mantis. It was just before Lao Sui's passing, in 1942, that Ma returned back to their village in Huiyang by boat and it was Ma Ming Sen alone who is responsible for Chu Gar being trained in Lao Sui's birthplace of Huiyang, Huizhou today. More of this story is to follow.

Let us now consider further a few notes of clarification as stated by Lao's family today:

- Wong Fook Go was a wandering medicine seller, not a monk as has been stated elsewhere previously.

- It is not known if Wong Fook Go called Chu Gar as Mantis.

- Lao Sui did call his kungfu as Chu Gar Mantis.

- Some in the original areas still only say Chu Gar Gao not Mantis.

- Lao Sui trained 4 years under his Master Wong from 1899-1903.

- Lao Sui went to Hong Kong in 1903 after 4 years of Chu Gar training.

- Lao started teaching Chu Gar in Hong Kong circa 1917 -18.

當劉水公開在香港傳授朱家螳螂拳後, 朱家螳螂拳開始蓬勃發展, 他有許多追隨多年情同骨肉的學生以及數百名拜於門下習藝的學生和再傳弟子。

最為親近他的人是他的兒子劉偉強, 女婿馬銘森和其他弟子包括楊壽, 朱渣五, 胡源, 葉喜, 朱冠華, 林華, 譚華, 譚照, 孫梓興和葉瑞等, 其中葉瑞師傅將習自劉水的武術傳之於世, 但冠以周家, 除此之外劉水仍稱他的武術為朱家螳螂, 今日 (2013 年) 在他的家鄉惠陽, 仍然稱他們的武術為朱家。

馬銘森三十歲時在惠陽老家娶劉水女兒為妻, 隨後循東江而下前往香港投奔劉水, 自1937年至1941年馬銘森一直在香港跟隨劉水學習朱家螳螂, 在劉水過世前 (1942年) 返回惠陽縣, 事實上在劉水故鄉, 馬銘森是唯一將劉水絕技帶回惠陽並在此落地生根的人 。

根據劉水留在惠陽老家後人的敘述, 讓我們重新審視並澄清下列幾個重點黃福高是游走四方的醫者, 而非像過往所稱的出家僧人。

究竟黃福高稱他所傳的武術為
朱家教或朱家螳螂, 今日無法查證。

劉水確曾稱他所傳的武術為朱家螳螂。

至今在發源地仍然只稱朱家教不言螳螂。

劉水追隨黃福高習藝四年 (1899年–1903年) 。

劉水得傳黃福高武藝後於1903年移居香港。

大約在1917年到1918年間劉水開始在香港公開教授朱家螳螂。

Chu Gar Mantis in Guangdong, China

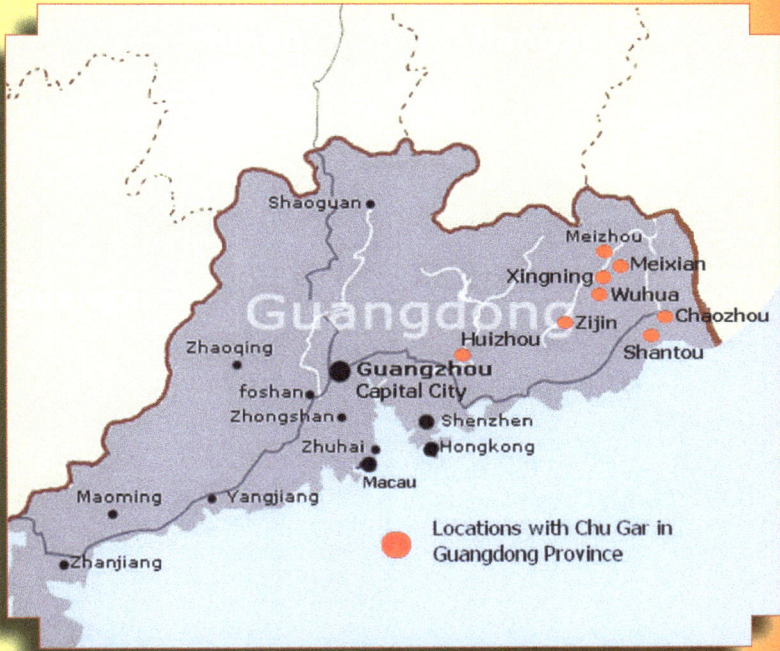

Chu Gar Gao - 朱家教 - Chu Family Creed

Zhu Jia Jiao is the correct pinyin for what
is commonly called Chu Gar Gao

Chu Gar Mantis - probably not named Mantis before Lao Sui

Chu Gar Mantis, Lao Sui Lineage, in China

- **Chu Ya Nan, 1st Generation Ancestor**

- **Wong Fook Go, 2nd Generation**

- **Lao Sui, 3rd Generation**

- **Ma Ming Sen, 4th Generation**

- **Current 5th generation includes:
  Sifus Ma Jiu Hua, Chen Jian Ming,
  Xie Tian Sheng, Lin Yun Yi and others**

27

朱家螳螂在中國廣東省

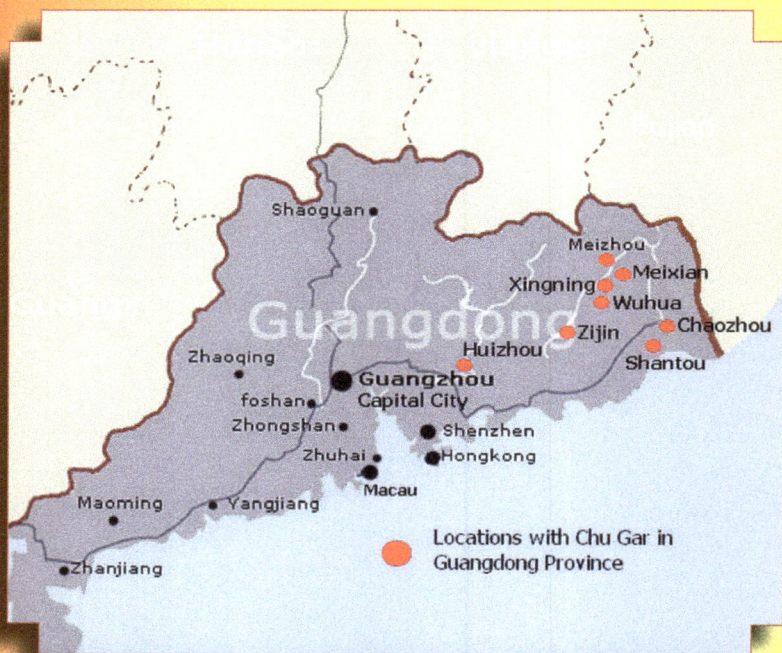

Locations with Chu Gar in Guangdong Province

朱家教常以 Chu Gar Gao
（粵語威妥瑪式拼音）或 Zhu Jia Jiao（漢語拼音）書寫

朱家螳螂拳一名始自劉水

惠州朱家螳螂拳劉水系族譜

朱亞南　創派祖師

黃福　高　二傳
劉水　三傳
馬銘森　四傳
五傳包括：
馬九華，陳建明，
謝添勝，林潤宇，
等等

Chu Jin, Son of Chu Ya Nan, in Boluo, Huizhou

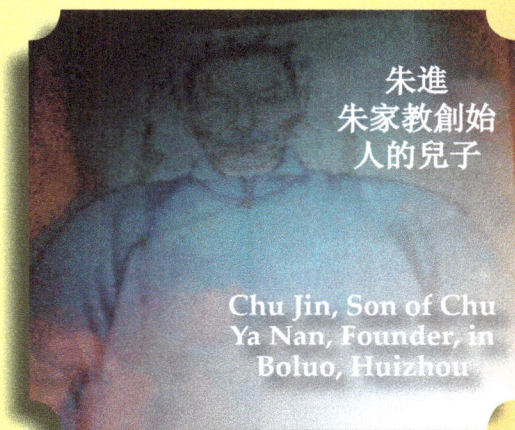

朱進
朱家教創始
人的兒子

Chu Jin, Son of Chu
Ya Nan, Founder, in
Boluo, Huizhou

Above: Chu Jin's image is retained by his grandson today in Boluo County. Chu Jin is the son of Chu Gar founder, Chu Ya Nan.

A number of stories exist about the founder Chu and his family.

Story 1

In the last years of the Ching Dynasty (circa 1912), Chu Huang Er left his home in Wuhua County, Guangdong and headed to Foshan City where martial arts were popular, especially Wing Chun. In Foshan, Chu started his own business buying and selling and trained kungfu diligently under the tutelage of a Hakka Sifu. In his later years, he returned back to Wuhua County where he decided to teach his kin and fellow villagers his martial art. Of all who learned from him, Chu Ya Nan was said to be the best.

Story 2

After the failure of the Taiping Heavenly Kingdom Rebellion, circa 1870, many of the rebel heroes congregated in the Meizhou, Jiaying area where Chu Gar Gao flourished under the leadership of Chu Ya Nan and became known as one of the 13 popular boxing styles of Guangdong. Thereafter Chu Gar Gao spread widely through the areas as shown on the aforementioned map.

Story 3

The Chu's were a rich family in the Wuhua area and lived a

29

朱亞南的兒子朱進在惠州市博羅縣

上圖為是由博羅縣朱進子孫所保留的朱進遺像，
朱進是朱家教創始人朱亞南的兒子。

關於朱亞南和他的家族存在著若干不同的軼聞。

故事 1

清王朝的最後一年(約西元 1912 年)，朱黃二, 離開廣東省五華縣家鄉，前往詠春拳最為流行的佛山鎮，開始他買賣並追隨客家師傅學習功夫。在他晚年時返回五華縣，教導家族子弟和同村村民他的武術，其中最為傑出的徒弟就是朱亞南。

故事 2

大約在 1870 年 太平天國叛亂，清朝平定太平天國之亂，許多太平天國的徒 ，其中不乏身懷絕藝之士，避禍於今日梅州嘉應一帶，其中朱家教在朱亞南的領導下，蓬勃發展成為廣東省十三名拳之一。此後朱家教廣泛傳於上述地圖上所示的區域。

故事 3

朱亞南出生五華地區一個富裕的家庭，過著悠閒的生活。朱亞南延請客家師傅劉廣才至他家教導功夫，並執以第子禮貢養於家中，劉廣才師傅將他畢生所學都傳給朱亞南，隨後朱亞南又傳給他的兒子朱進，朱進藝成後浪跡於粵東，四處教導朱家教功夫及行醫。

據說在上世紀20年代，朱進常背著采藥籃上插一支旗，上面書寫著(專精修補破拳頭)，有一次在汕頭震邦街附近的客棧中，客棧老闆熊長慶也是習武之人，看到朱進回答說：如果一個人功夫好當然不需要修理，但如果功夫爛，我可以修復它！熊長慶聽聞後大膽地要求朱進證明給他看。

朱回答你是主，我是客，客隨主便。於是熊長慶在大廳中演示他的功夫，他的動作有如一陣風，大廳四處塵土飛揚併發出如雷巨聲。

leisurely life. And so, Chu Ya Nan sought out a Hakka Sifu named Liu Guang Cai and invited him into the Chu family home to live and teach kungfu. Liu Sifu accepted and lived many years passing all his teaching of Chu Gar Gao to Chu Ya Nan, who enjoyed hard training. In turn, Chu Ya Nan transmitted all he had to his son Chu Jin, who became a mysterious wanderer travelling throughout eastern Guangdong teaching kungfu and healing people as a "dit da" herbal doctor.

It is said that Chu Jin as he wandered about in the 1920s, carried a medicine basket over his shoulder with two flags mounted on top. The two flags had written on them, "fix and repair broken boxing." Once, when passing an Inn in Shantou City, Zhenbang Street, the big boss, a martial artist by the name of Xiong Changqing, saw Chu Jin's flags and said to him, "you must be exaggerating your martial skill" to which Chu Jin replied, "if someone is good, then no repair is needed, but if the kungfu is broken, I can repair it." Xiong thinking it brazen asked, "Then why not demonstrate it?"

Chu replied, "You are the host here, I am the guest, etiquette states you first." And so, Xiong Changqing, in the lobby of the Inn, immediately began stirring dust by a whirlwind of motion and deafening sounds! It turns out his kungfu was good! Afterwards he asked Chu Jin, "pray let us do have a look at your repair work now." Chu Jin replied, "I will show you a little, but afterwards you may not ask me to pay for damages I cause to your lobby floor." Xiong, the Inn Keeper, thought to himself, "I have trained kungfu many years on this floor without damage, what concern have I over you?" And so he prompted Chu Jin to carry on.

Chu Jin played a round of a Chu Gar form in which his iron steps left the flooring broken and in disrepair. Xiong Changqing was greatly surprised and exclaimed loudly that he had not previously seen such a kungfu expert! Xiong quickly knelt before Chu Jin and asked to learn Chu's boxing. And so, for three years Chu Jin remained in Shantou City and taught Xiong all he could learn. Afterwards, Chu left the Shantou area and no one there had any news of him or where he may have gone.

Later in the 1930s, Xiong, the Inn Keeper, heard that someone was teaching Chu Gar Gao near the Shantou bus terminal and immediately went to investigate. It turned out to be another student of the wandering Chu Jin, by the name of Wong Chun Keung. Wong taught many years there and had a number of good students, and chief among them was Zhong Tingfang.

事實上熊長慶的功夫已非尋常！他問朱進可否讓我們開開眼界啊？朱進回答說：我會讓你看到，但你不可要我賠償你的大廳地板，客棧老闆認為到自己已經在此大廳練武多年，而地板絲毫無損，不信朱進會造成什麼損害，於是他一再敦促朱進演練。

當朱進表演朱家教套路時，他每一步都將地板踏的碎裂，熊長慶很吃驚地大聲嚷道他從來沒見過這種功夫！熊長慶立即跪在朱進面前，請朱進收他為徒。朱進留在汕頭三年教導熊長慶他所有的功夫，之後朱進離開汕頭不知去向。

稍後熊長慶聽說有人在汕頭客運站附近開館教朱家教，登門造訪才發現武館師傅黃振強也是游走四方朱進的學生，黃師傅在汕頭開館多年教了很多學生，其中最出名的是鐘庭芳。

在上世紀30年代鐘庭芳在香港靠拉人力車為生，有一次看到外國人和賣水果的人爭執，外國人砸爛中國人的水果攤並揍了中國人一頓，鐘親眼目睹外國人欺壓中國人痛歐外國人。

香港警署通緝鐘庭芳想抓他歸案，他潛逃回廣東省汕頭，靠同鄉掩護隱匿了一段時間後，他易名在汕頭開了一間理髮店。

偶然鐘庭芳逛街時聽說朱進的學生黃振強教導一種絕佳的武術叫做朱家教，所以鐘庭芳登門求教並說黃師傅，如果我不能擊敗你，我會拜你為師，但如果我打敗你，你必須對我磕頭。商定後，黃振強總是輕鬆地化解他每一次的攻擊，於是鐘庭芳不得不跪下拜黃振強為師。黃振強和鐘庭芳師徒倆配合良好，在黃振強的教導下鐘庭芳掌握了朱家教的精髓，在某段時間裡，他們同時各自開館授徒，最後鐘庭芳的傳承被稱為汕頭(鳳凰爪朱家教)。鐘庭芳在1917年出生，1992年去世。

故事 4

傳說朱家教創於福建省九連山的南少林寺，然而這傳說據說是為了要隱藏其真實的發源地—位於東江源頭的江西竹林寺，隱居於竹林寺禪宗和尚觀看螳螂搏鬥而悟得螳螂拳，在他晚年，將螳螂拳傳給第子林博官，

林博官的妻子吳氏也來自於武術世家，自幼耳濡目染，

The history of Zhong is, as a young man, he worked in Hong Kong pulling a rickshaw. Once he saw a foreigner and a fruit seller having an argument. The foreigner destroyed the Chinese fruit seller's stall and gave the seller a beating. Zhong having witnessed that felt the foreigner was unjust and therefore, even before learning kungfu, took action against the foreigner and beat him severely.

As a result the Police department wanted to catch Zhong for questioning, but he fled back to the Shantou area in Guangdong, where his town's folk kept him hidden for a time. Eventually, he changed his name and opened a barber shop, staying in Shantou.

By chance, Zhong was out and about one day and heard Wong Chu Keung, the student of Chu Jin, was teaching an excellent boxing called Chu Gar Gao near the Shantou bus terminal. And so, Zhong sought him out and said, "Wong Sifu, if I cannot beat your kungfu, then I will join you, but if I defeat you, then you must kowtow to me." Agreed upon, several times Zhong tried to best Wong who easily thwarted his every attempt. And so, Zhong had to kneel and accept Wong Chun Keung as his teacher. Wong and Zhong were a good match, teacher with student, and Zhong excelled at Chu Gar Gao under Wong's tutelage. In time, they both were teaching and eventually Zhong's teaching became known as "Phoenix Claw Chu Gar" of Shantou City. Zhong was born in 1917 and passed in 1992.

Story 4

Chu Gar was created at the southern Shaolin Temple on "Jiulian" Mountain in Fujian Province. However, this was said to be a ruse to cover its origination at the source of the East River in Jiangxi (Kwongsai) Province at the Bamboo Forest Temple. It was at this Bamboo Forest Temple that a Zen monk, late in his years, passed the Art he had created by watching a mantis, to his disciple Lin Bo Guan. Lin's wife, Wu Xueshi, came from a family whose kungfu employed the "like Chinese character ding but not ding" and "like Chinese character 8 but not 8" footwork without making a sound, cat and panther fist skills collectively known as dragon fist, sinking the chest, rounding the back and inch force tactics. Lin and his wife combined skills and taught many students but none learned in-depth or well.

At this time, the person named Chu Ya Nan was on the run and was wanted for his anti-Ching Dynasty activities. And so he took

其家傳武術立馬(丁 不 丁，八 不 八)行步無聲和貓及豹拳手法統稱為龍形拳，其身形行含胸圓背，注重寸勁。林博官和他的妻子整合所有武術並以之教過許多學生，但始終沒有學生出類拔萃。

此時有一名為朱亞南的人因從事反清活動而被通緝，逃至竹林寺為老和尚收容，老和尚將螳螂拳傳給朱亞南，因他年事已高，故而委託林博官繼續教導朱亞南。

朱亞南在林博官的諒諒教導下，悟得老和尚螳螂拳的真諦，因朱亞南被通緝，必須不斷逃移，最後定居在廣東省五華縣，在居地公開教授他的功夫，並以他的姓氏命名，稱之為朱家教。

朱亞南收了許多第子以繼承他反清的志業，其中兩位黃姓門徒（黃進修和黃和策）遠赴東南亞包括今天的馬來西亞和新加坡，在吉隆坡他們公開與各方的武術家在擂臺上比武，其間黃進修曾搏剎了一個當地名叫邱太虎的武術家。

因此雙黃在當地聲名大噪，許多人爭先投入其門下，有一位來自於東莞的劉才官也入門成為第子，劉才官也引進盤龍棍和十八手到朱家教的系統中，回國後劉才官加入太平天軍，退休後隱居於一座修道院中，他的學生和再傳在20世紀初將朱家教傳到福建、廣東、廣西和東南亞地區。

中國劉水家族的故事

無論是在香港或中國對劉水所傳的武術均稱之為朱家教或朱家螳螂拳，事實上直到劉水在香港過世後，在香港才出現(周家)的名稱。

今天在中國劉水的故鄉，人們仍稱其所遺留的武術為朱家教或朱家螳螂，今年來劉水後人更親往朱家教的發源地—廣東省興寧市尋根。

劉水的師傅黃福高，大約在1899年曆經130英里遙遠的路程，從興寧到達惠陽縣，他可能一路奔波馬不停蹄，也可能游走四方，沿路醫治病患和販賣藥物。

refuge at the Bamboo Forest Temple where Lin Bo Guan's master, the Zen Monk, was taking refuge. The Zen Monk seeing Chu Ya Nan was quite capable taught him kungfu and later sent him to Lin Bo Guan to learn all.

Under Lin's tutelage, Chu Ya Nan learned the secrets of the Zen Monk's Mantis boxing. As Chu was wanted and hunted by the Ching court, he kept on the move but eventually settled in Wuhua County, Guangdong. There he took residence and taught widely the kungfu of the Bamboo Forest Temple, calling it by his family's surname, Chu Gar Gao.

Chu Ya Nan accepted many disciples who carried on the anti-Ching rebellion. Two of his disciples surnamed Wong (Wong Jing Shou and Wong He Che) carried Chu Gar Gao into the islands of Southeast Asia, including Malaysia and Singapore. In Kuala Lumpur, they engaged in "Lei-Tai" bouts or matches on a raised platform and Wong Jing Shou killed a local boxer named Qiu Taihu.

As a result, Wong's name grew in fame and many people sought him to become disciples. One such person named Liu Cai Guan introduced "Panlong (dragon) staff and 18 hands to the Chu Gar. Liu was instrumental in the Taiping Uprising and later retired to a monastery. Many people also sought him and his students further spread Chu Gar Gao to Fujian, Guangdong, Guangxi and Southeast Asia at the turn of the 20th century.

Story as told by Lao Sui's Family in China

The Art that Lao Sui trained and taught in China and Hong Kong has always been called Chu Gar Gao or Chu Gar Mantis. It wasn't until after his death in Hong Kong that the Art became confused as Chow Gar (Zhou Gar).

In China today, the Art is still called Chu Gar Gao or either Chu Gar Mantis. In recent years, the descendants of Lao Sui travelled to the original areas near Xingning City from whence Chu Gar came to Lao's village in Huiyang District, Huizhou.

When Wong Fook Go, circa 1899, travelled the 130 miles or so from Xingning to Lao Sui's hometown he would likely have been on horseback for several days or longer, maybe even stopping here and there in many villages as he treated patients and sold his medicine.

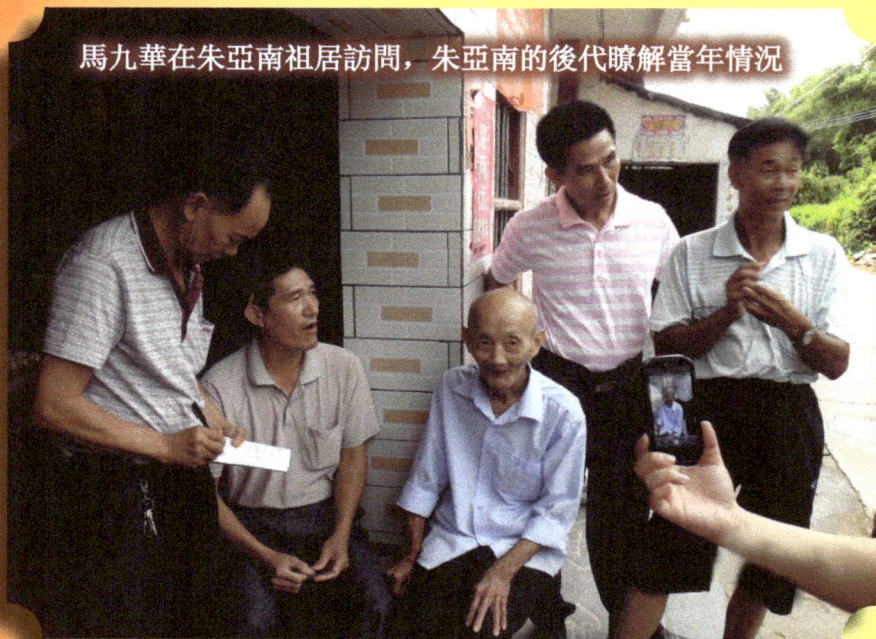

馬九華在朱亞南祖居訪問，朱亞南的後代瞭解當年情況

Ma Jiuhua and other brothers from Lao Sui's home travelled to the Xingning, Wuhua areas to meet with Chu Gar founder, Chu Ya Nan's, descendants who are still living and visit his ancestral home.

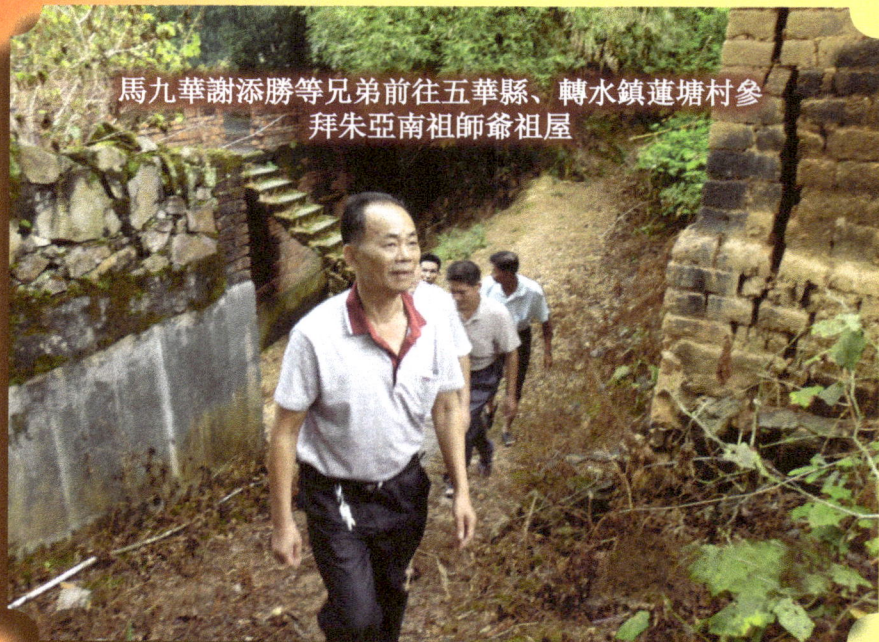

馬九華謝添勝等兄弟前往五華縣、轉水鎮蓮塘村參
拜朱亞南祖師爺祖屋

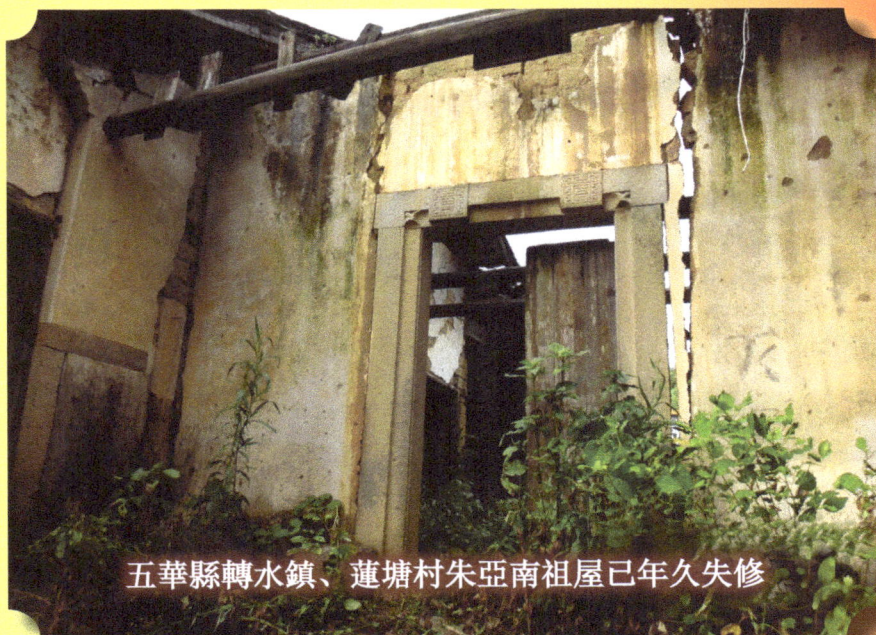

五華縣轉水鎮、蓮塘村朱亞南祖屋已年久失修

The ancestral home of Chu Gar founder, Chu Ya Nan, still stands in Meizhou City, Wuhua County, Zhuanshui Town, (转水镇), although as seen in these photographs, it is in complete disrepair.

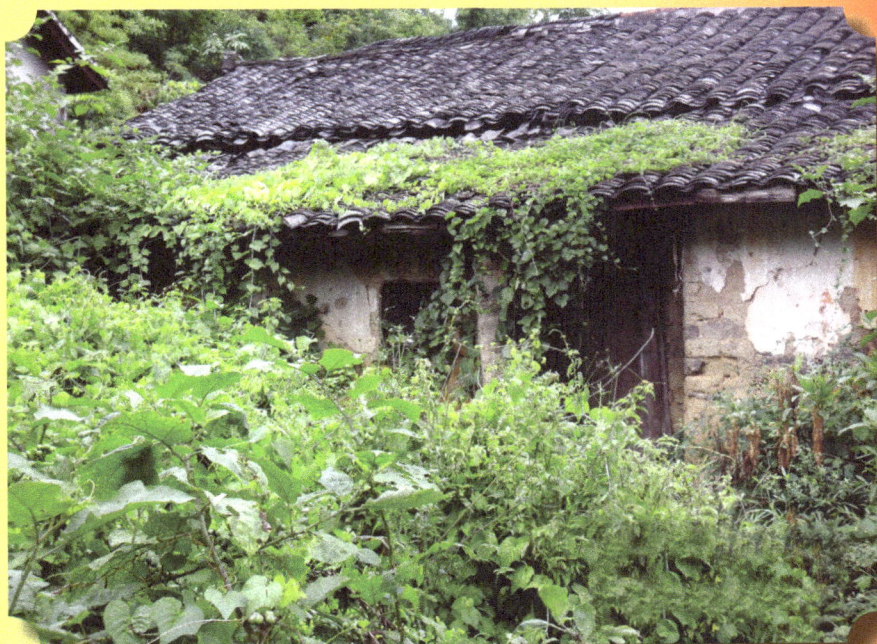

馬偉波外曾孫和謝添勝審視朱家教創始人朱亞南文物《劍》

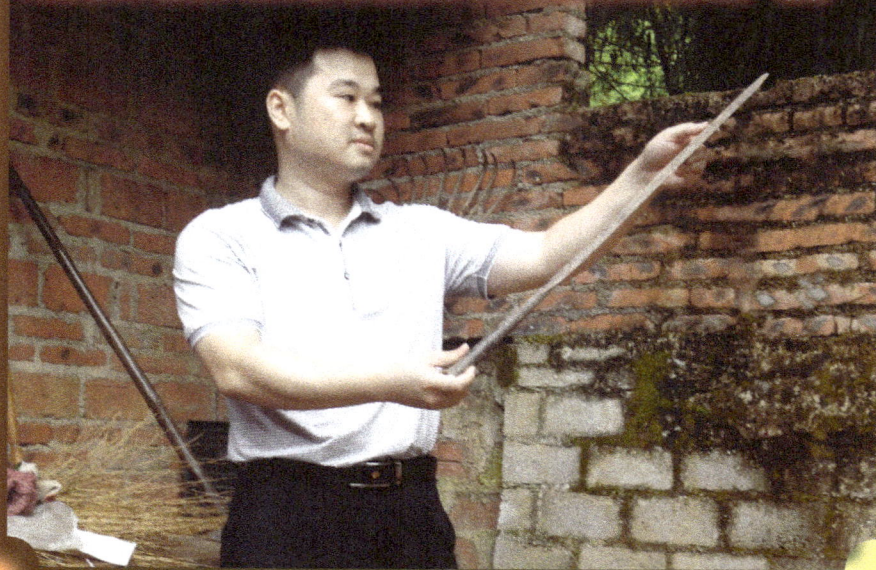

Above: Ma Weibo, great grandson of Lao Sui, examines Chu Gar founder, Chu Ya Nan's, artifacts. Below: Xie Tiansheng Sifu shows the sword that Chu Gar Mantis founder Chu Ya Nan carried.

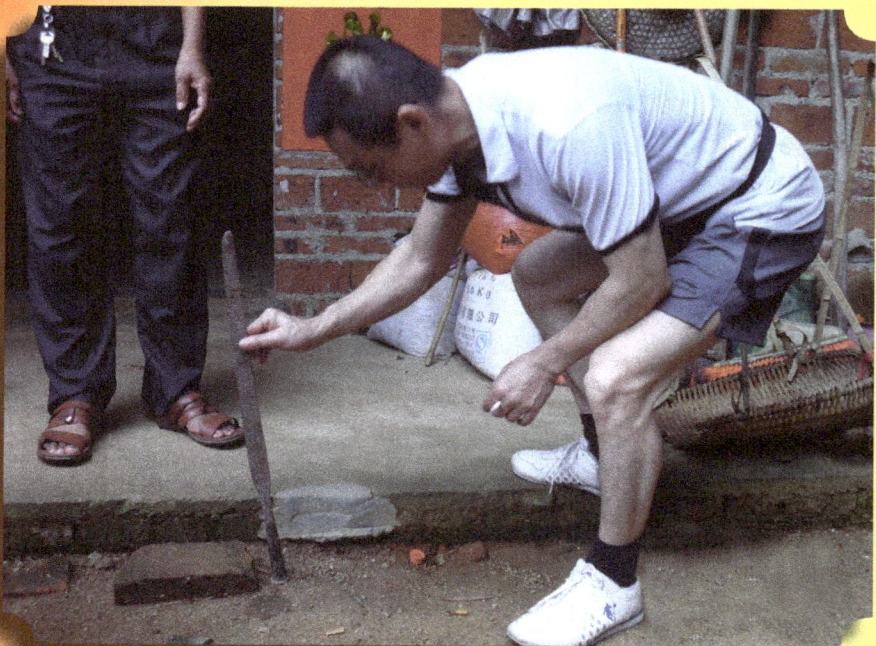

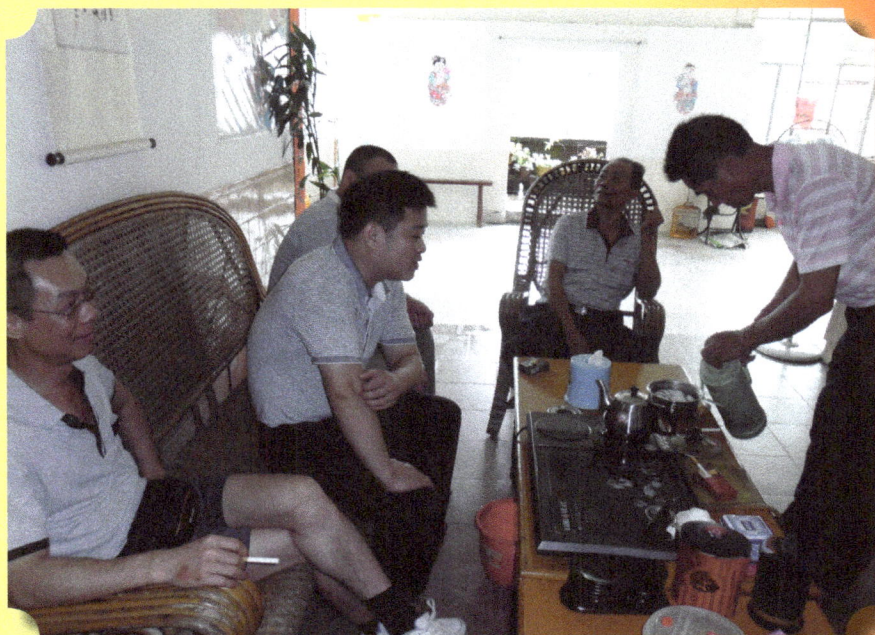

These two photos show the family and students of Lao Sui returning to the very root of Chu Gar and visiting with the relatives of founder Chu Ya Nan. The woman centered was the host of Chu's family.

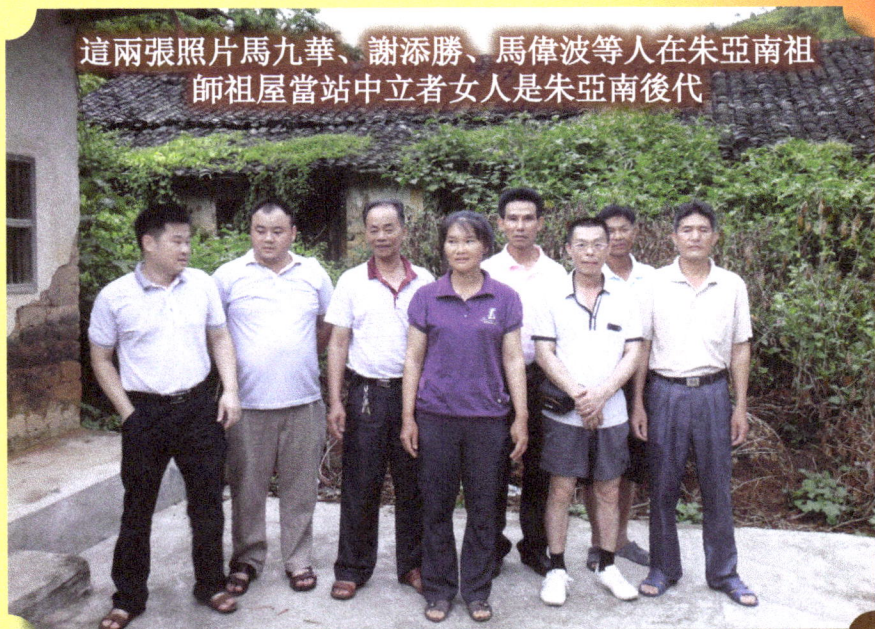

這兩張照片馬九華、謝添勝、馬偉波等人在朱亞南祖師祖屋當站中立者女人是朱亞南後代

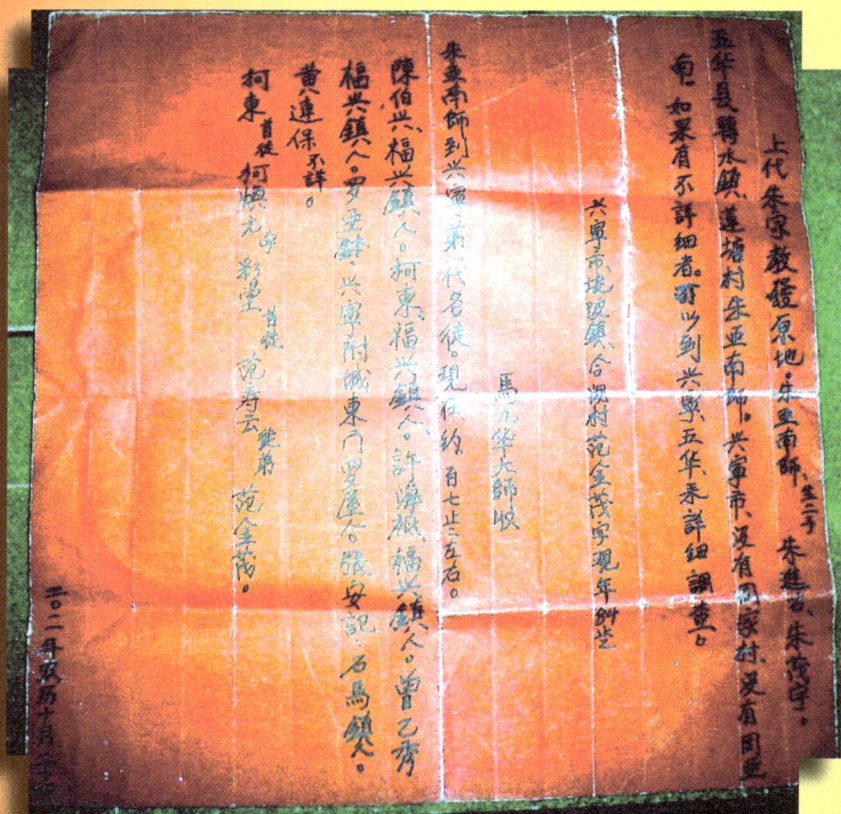

上面照片是：

馬九華、謝添勝等人去興甯尋找朱亞南祖屋時，一個朱家教後代叫范金茂（84歲）師傅寫給馬九華的信，介紹當地朱亞南在興甯的名徒.

回顾

我们可以清楚瞭解朱家螳螂拳的历史与太平天国和白莲教秘密会党的纠葛，他们主要的诉求就是反清复明。这不是在讲古，而是发生于19世纪80年代到二十世纪初的史实。南方螳螂拳定型大约是近150年的事，我们也知道创始人朱亚南的儿子朱进的后代仍居住在博罗县，朱亚南的族人也可在五华县转水镇找到。

在这一章中我们已经追随朱家教的起源和上世纪30年代的传承。在这下文中，我们将介绍朱家教在刘水故乡由他的女婿马铭森延续的传承。

請繼續閱讀，瞭解更多。

Photo left: Fan Jianmao, martial art historian aged 84, lives in the Wuhua area and has written a letter to Ma Jiuhua Sifu and the pupils of Lao Sui in the Huiyang District stating that Chu Ya Nan, founder of Chu Gar Mantis' ancestral home is in Zhuanshui Town, that no Chow (Zhou) Gar, Chow An Nam, or Chow Gar Gao exists, and he extends an invitation for anyone who thinks otherwise to visit and see for themselves.

Reflections

We can see that the history of Chu may be connected with the Taiping Rebellion and the White Lotus Secret Societies which were involved with "Fan Ching Fuk Ming" or overthrow the Ching and restore the Ming. This was not in antiquity but was as late as 1880s to 1915. Southern Mantis styles are barely 150 years old as we know them today. The great grandson several generations down line of Chu Jin, the son of founder Chu Ya Nan, lives in Boluo, Huizhou today and the descendants of founder Chu Ya Nan are still living in Chu's hometown of Zhuanshui in Wuhua County.

In this chapter we've revisited the origins and transmission of Chu Gar as recently as the 1930s. In the following pages, we'll visit the transmission from Lao Sui, in the late 1930s, and Chu Gar's return to Lao Sui's hometown by his Son-in-law, Ma Ming Sen, in the 1940s.

Read on to know more of this.

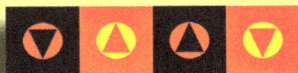

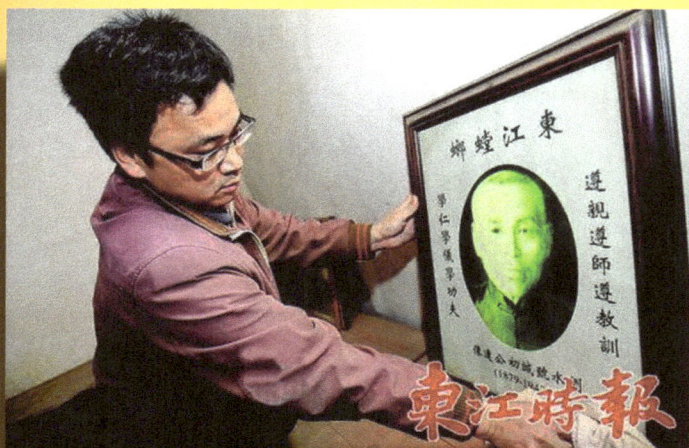

Lao Jian Chang, 38, holds the memorial photograph of his grand uncle Lao Sui, 2013, Huiyang, Huizhou

Chu Gar Mantis School of Lao Sui

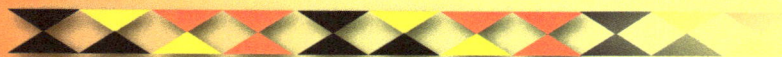

Hong Yuen Village Conceals the Southern School of Mantis Boxing in the Home of Lao Sui

劉水傳朱家螳螂

香園村暗藏南派螳螂拳"劉屋洋樓"原來有段古

東江流域的民眾自古尚武好義，在惠州產生過東江龍形拳、李家拳、白眉拳等蜚聲中外的拳種，湧現出林耀桂、李義、張禮泉等著名拳師。2月16日，"惠州邊界行"採訪組在蘆洲鎮香園村發現，香園村暗藏一種名叫南派螳螂拳的拳種。仿照螳螂的身形馬步、沉肩墮肘懸吊索三箭拳及吞胸拔背的筲箕背鐵尺腰......剛柔並濟的螳螂拳，讓人大飽眼福。

Since ancient times, the people of the Dongjiang East River basin have been skilled in warfare. In Huizhou City, there is the Dongjiang Dragon Fist boxing, Li Gar, and White Eyebrow boxing, which emerged from the famous masters named Lin Yaogui, Li Yi, and Zhang Liquan. On February 16, 2012, an interview by the East River Times Newspaper found a hidden faction of Southern Mantis boxing in Luchou Town, Hong Yuen Village. Modeled on a mantis' movements, boxers learn firm steps, soft and hard power, sink the chest and round the back, iron waist, and Three Step Arrow boxing. It is a feast for the eyes.

The Southern Mantis School third-generation descendant, Lao Sui, flourished in Hong Kong in the 1930s. However, as recently as 2008, the disciples and family members of Lao Sui in Huizhou, China, Lao's hometown, discovered that by accident Southern Praying Mantis in Hong Kong had divided into two factions, Chow Gar and Chu Gar. Accordingly, further research was conducted in the location where this Southern Mantis originated, Meizhou, China. It was discovered that Chow and Chu pronunciation in Meizhou Hakka dialect are very similar, but the original ancestor in China is named Chu (Zhu) Ya Nan. Chu's descendants still live in this area. Without question, the name of Lao Sui's Mantis legacy in China and his hometown is Chu Gar from Chu Ya Nan.

However, to avoid confusion we can say that the whole of Southern Mantis may be collectively referred to today as Dongjiang (East River) Southern Praying Mantis without the distinction of Chow or Chu.

Lao Sui trains Chu Gar four years under his Master, Wong Fook Go

Today in Luchou Town, Hong Yuen Village, remains a two story brick and wood home that was built by Lao Sui circa 1936. The second floor has a large balcony with peaches, bats, and other sculptures on thick wooden eaves which are engraved with auspicious Chinese words like "lucky." The double door main entrance is still solid and steady. There is a story of the martial artist, Lao Sui, behind this old building which is still the family home of his descendants today. (Refer to page 143.)

南派螳螂拳第三代傳人劉水將該拳種在香港發揚光大。不過，讓南派螳螂拳惠州弟子們意外的是，該拳種在香港有周家和朱家兩派之分。據他們前往五華縣轉水鎮蓮塘村考證，周和朱兩字在梅州客家話中極為相似，南派螳螂拳的宗師應為朱亞南。他們因此計畫為南派螳螂拳正名，取消周、朱之分，統稱為南派東江螳螂拳。

劉水20歲拜師學螳螂拳24歲赴港開館授徒

據香港出版的拳譜、劉水弟子葉瑞編寫的《東江螳螂拳》記載，時際清末，劉水避亂至香港，因技高德偉，遐邇知名，桃李遍港九，從學者無數。

在蘆洲鎮香園村，有一棟民國時期的兩層磚木結構小洋樓，二樓有寬大的陽臺，翹角的屋簷上有壽桃、蝙蝠等雕塑點綴，還刻有"吉祥"、"如意"等字樣，條石砌成的大門顯得堅實、沉穩。這棟樓被當地人稱為"劉屋洋樓"，在舊屋原址上修建，已有70年歷史，背後隱藏著一位武術家的故事。

這位武術家的名字叫劉水，號初誠，1879年生於香園村。劉水自幼愛好無數，年少時習馬家拳，還自創了劉水棍術，20歲時已以拳棍聞名鄉里。蘆洲與觀音閣隔著東江相望，當時，蘆洲人常乘船到觀音閣鎮趁圩。每到觀音閣鎮圩日，劉水喜歡去逛一逛，尋找高手比武。

彼時，南派螳螂拳第二代傳人、興甯人黃福高適逢到觀音閣行醫賣藥，見劉水是一個習武的好苗子，就對劉水說他的功夫很好，可惜還未到上乘之境。年少氣盛的劉水要求與黃福高比武。幾個回合下來，劉水就被黃福高制伏。劉水當即跪拜黃福高為師，跟著師傅學南派螳螂拳，當時劉水只有20歲。

經過黃福高4年的精心指導，劉水練就一身過硬的南派螳螂拳，還學會了刀槍、跌打醫術，成為南派螳螂拳第三代傳人。1903年，24歲的劉水到香港發展，在香港九龍開館授徒。據香港出版的拳譜、劉水弟子葉瑞編寫的《東江螳螂拳》記載，時際清末，劉水避亂至香港，因技高德偉，遐邇知名，桃李遍港九，從學者無數。

Lao Sui's original name was Lao Cheng and he was born in 1879, in the aforementioned Hong Yuen Village. Since childhood Lao had a love of martial arts and trained all kinds of local Hakka kungfu. By the age of 20, he was quite famous for his staff skills and readily taught others boxing. Just across the East River was the Goddess of Mercy Pavilion (Guanyinge) and the Luchou people often crossed over by boat on their way to the market. On festive days, Lao Sui would go around seeking martial art masters to have a contest.

On one such occasion, the second generation Southern Mantis descendant, Wong Fook Go from Xingning City, happened to be at the Goddess of Mercy Pavilion practicing medicine and selling drugs. There he observed Lao Sui's kungfu but said that it appeared good but wasn't really useful. And so, the young and fit Lao Sui engaged Wong in several rounds of boxing, each of which Lao was easily subdued. Immediately Lao recognized Wong had superior skill and kowtowed to become Wong Fook Go's pupil when he was 20 years old.

After four years of careful guidance, Lao Sui had become an excellent Southern Mantis boxer and also had learned the skills of knives and guns, bone setting, and medicine and became known as the third-generation descendant of Chu Gar Southern Praying Mantis. In 1903, the 24 year old Lao went to Hong Kong and never returned to his birthplace.

Lao Sui Builds a Home But Does Not Return to His Roots

In 1936 Lao Sui was over the age of 50, and had the idea of returning to his roots. So he asked a friend to bring money back to Huizhou to build a home. It took more than four years to complete construction. Today, his family still lives in this house.

After arriving in Hong Kong, Lao Sui taught Chu Gar boxing and his younger brother, Lao Fu Yuan studied medicine. After Fu Yuan completed his study, he went back to their family home in Luchou and passed down his knowledge to his family. In 2013, Lao Jian Chang, the grandson of Lao Fu Yuan, has inherited the mantle and continues practicing medicine in the home Lao Sui had constructed in 1936.

建"劉屋洋樓"無奈落葉難歸根

劉屋洋樓"建于1936年，當時劉水年逾50，有落葉歸根的想法，當時在香港托朋友帶錢回來。這房子一建就是4年多。

雖然劉水離開家鄉，但對故鄉蘆洲的思念及與親友的聯繫交往卻從未斷絕。

劉水在香港設館教拳師，他的弟弟劉富元曾到香港跟其學醫，得其真傳，後回到觀音閣、蘆洲等地，成為一代名醫。而今，劉富元的孫子劉振強繼承其衣缽，繼續在香園村行醫，繼續居住在"劉屋洋樓"裡。

"劉屋洋樓"建于1936年，當時劉水年逾50，有葉落歸根的想法，當時在香港托朋友帶錢回來。這房子一建就是4年多，1941年竣工時，日軍已全面入侵中國，香港淪陷。

劉水曾經返回家鄉，但回至深圳時身體不適，又因為戰亂交通阻塞，只好折返香港。劉水遺留下來的兩首詩，一首可以看出他當時的思鄉之情："虛度光陰數十年，今春首采假居先；歸家心急如星火，斷絕交通恨不前；欲圖冒險回桑梓，中途兵災又掛牽；雖是暫時羈此地，誠驚故我亦依然。"

另一首則看出劉水歸鄉無望後的失望之情："浪跡江湖覓食多，平生志願望蹉跎；香園歸隱非吾願，六親情切付東河。大地既無干淨土，宗邦禦敵動干戈。從今勘破紅塵界，萬念皆空一夢柯。"

思鄉心切的劉水，積慮于心，1942年在香港抱憾去世，享年64歲，離鄉30載未歸，魂散香江。

弟子馬銘森在惠收徒傳授螳螂拳
馬銘森稱呼劉水為"同年爺"。1937年，30歲的馬銘森到香港拜劉水學武，一學就是5年，練就一身功夫，並于1941年返鄉。

雖然劉水沒有在惠州教授過弟子，但因為香園村人馬銘森

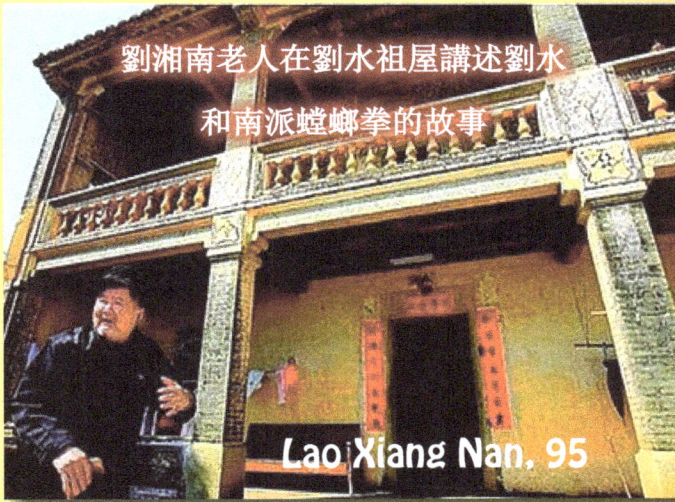

劉湘南老人在劉水祖屋講述劉水
和南派螳螂拳的故事

Lao Xiang Nan, 95

Lao Xiang Nan, 95, plays Chu Gar Mantis at the home Lao Sui financed but never was able to see. Lao Xiang Nan is the son of Lao Fu Yuan, Lao Sui's brother.

Once, Lao Sui decided to return home but upon reaching Shenzhen, just inside China's border, could not go further due to the Japanese invading China. Travelling wasn't easy and Lao's health had also taken a turn for the worse. Although within days of reaching his home, he decided to turn back to Hong Kong.

Later on he wrote some lines of poetry expressing his feelings of being homesick. (Refer to the translations on page 156 - 157.) Lao actively kept his family in mind until his passing in 1942, at age 64. He was never able to return home. His final resting place is in Hong Kong today.

Disciple Ma Ming Sen Returns Chu Gar Mantis to Huizhou

In Lao Sui's village, the Ma family was the Lao family's next door neighbor. The Ma and Lao families still live next door to each other in 2013. Their families are related by marriage as well. It was Ma Ming Sen who married Lao Sui's daughter. In 1937, the 30 year old Ma Ming Sen went to Hong Kong to learn Southern Mantis from Lao Sui. There he trained five years before returning back to their hometown, Huiyang, in 1941.

Lao Sui left for Hong Kong in 1903 and never returned to his hometown in China. It is because of his Son-in-law, Ma Ming Sen,

赴港學武，使得南派螳螂拳得以在惠州傳承。

據馬銘森的兒子、今年71歲的馬九華介紹，他的祖父與劉水是同齡結拜兄弟，馬銘森稱呼劉水為〝同年爺〞。1937年，30歲的馬銘森到香港拜劉水學武，一學就是5年，練就一身功夫，並于1941年返鄉。

令人疑惑的是，馬銘森在回來的二三十年間，幾乎沒有向外人展露過武功。〝父親回鄉後，歷經抗戰和解放戰爭，建國後又歷經特殊的政治環境，這也許是他未展露武功的根源.〞馬九華說，到1962年，他21歲的時候，馬銘森才偶爾教他一兩招螳螂拳鍛煉身體。

直至陳建明出現，馬銘森身懷絕技的秘密才被大家所知。1957年出生的陳建明，從小就喜歡舞刀弄槍，其父親當時在蘆洲鎮供銷社工作，打聽到馬銘森會功夫。1972年，陳建明拜馬銘森為師。後來，馬銘森在蘆洲鎮以及觀音閣鎮一帶也收了一些徒弟，觀音閣鎮人謝添勝就是其中之一。馬銘森每到觀音閣鎮時，都會到謝添勝家教他打拳。

1984年，77歲的馬銘森應邀到水口的一家武館當師傅，收了70多個徒弟，但真正學成者極少。1996年，90歲高齡的馬銘森在故里去世。

馬九華說，馬銘森屬於南派螳螂拳第四代傳人，該拳在惠弟子基本師承馬銘森。

惠州第子去五華縣轉水鎮蓮塘村考證祖師爺姓名

馬九華、謝添勝等人去興甯五華縣朱亞南老家考證，證實朱家教創始人是朱亞南、不是周亞南、所以劉水宗師傳受下來的應是朱家螳螂。

近些年，隨著武術運動的勃興，各種拳派尋根問祖熱也在興起。〝劉屋洋樓〞曾接待來自五湖四海的南派螳螂拳弟子，這些弟子們，均尊稱劉水為〞一代宗師〞。

與此同時，南派螳螂拳在惠州的傳人，也開始了尋根之

Sifu Chen Jian Ming

2009年

陳建明師傅接受惠州日報採訪時的專訪報導朱家螳螂拳

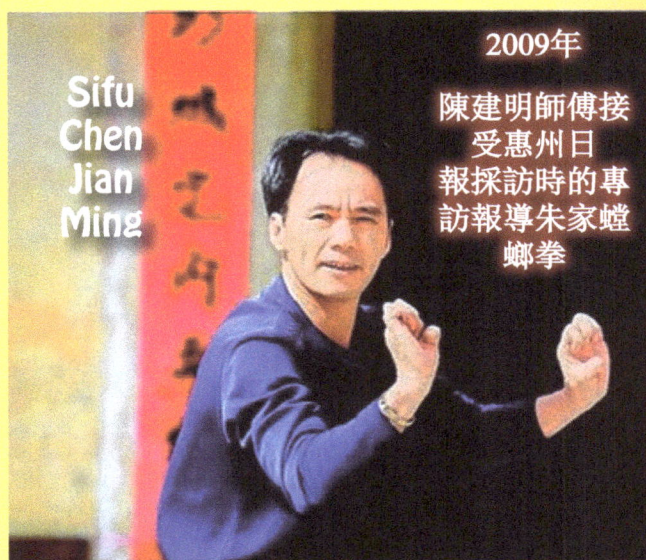

Chen Jian Ming, 55, is a leader of Chu Gar Mantis in Lao Sui's hometown today. He is the chief pupil of Lao Sui's Son-in-law, Ma Ming Sen.

that Chu Gar exists in Lao Sui's hometown today.

According to Ma Ming Sen's son, 71 year old Ma Jiuhua (cover of this book), his grandfather and Lao Sui, being village neighbors, were sworn brothers of the same age.

Ma Jiuhua said it was puzzling that for some years after returning from Hong Kong, his father, Ma Ming Sen, never showed or talked about learning Chu Gar Mantis from Lao Sui. It was the time of the Anti-Japanese War and the War of Liberation, and a special political environment existed, so perhaps the elder Ma did not expose his martial art for fear of persecution. Ma Jiuhua states that in 1962, when he was 21 years old, his father Ma Ming Sen only occasionally taught him twelve strokes Mantis boxing workouts.

Until Chen Jianming appeared in 1972, it was a great secret, in Lao Sui's home village, that Ma Ming Sen was a master of Chu Gar Mantis Kungfu. Chen Jianming was born in 1957, and his family was from Luchou town. As a boy, Chen trained Li Gar, Dragon and many kinds of village boxing. By accident he overheard a friend of his father talking about Ma Ming Sen's Chu Gar Mantis and so he travelled the long distance by small boat on the East River to ask Ma Ming Sen to teach him. Ma refused. Persistent, Chen returned many times by riding a bicycle more than 3 hours each time to petition Ma Sifu. Each time Ma refused. But one day, Ma spotted the young Chen Jian Ming playing kungfu and recognized

旅。2008年，馬九華等10多名師兄弟前往香港九龍拜會劉水嫡傳弟子葉瑞、鄭運等人。不過，讓馬九華等人困惑的是，在香港，由劉水發揚光大的南派螳螂拳都冠以〞東江〞之名，但卻分為周家和朱家兩拳派。

馬九華估計，這應該不是劉水弟子故意另立門戶，而可能是音誤。按照粵語發音，周和朱兩字發言極易分別，但五華客家話中的周和朱讀音難以辨別，基本是同一種讀音。馬九華認為，南派螳螂拳前三代均是客家人，有可能將周和朱混淆並傳播，造成了今日的分歧。按照葉瑞的資訊，南派螳螂拳的創始人應為周亞南，廣東興甯周家村人；而按照鄭運的理解，應為朱亞南，廣東五華人。到底孰對孰錯？

去年11月，馬九華等人前往五華興甯，遍尋興甯也找不到周家村。後來，他們又到了梅州五華，在五華轉水鎮蓮塘村找到了朱亞南的身份資訊和習拳經歷。

原來，朱亞南正是南派螳螂拳的祖師爺，于清朝中葉、200多年前到福建南少林追隨禪隱大師學習南少林拳，目睹螳螂與雀相鬥，創出螳螂拳。為了區別北方的螳螂拳，遂將其命名為南派螳螂拳。出寺後，朱亞南到東江一帶傳授給客家弟子，黃福高便是其一。

為了證明亞南姓〞朱〞而非〞周〞，南派螳螂拳在興甯的第四傳人范金茂去年11月29日寫字條給馬九華，稱只有五華縣轉水鎮蓮塘村朱亞南，興甯市沒有周家村，沒有周亞南，如有不詳細者可到興甯、五華來調查。

南派螳螂拳祖師爺的名字終於水落石出，馬九華如釋重負。他把這些考究成果都展覽在他自己設立的香園村南派螳螂拳陳列館裡。他和其他師兄弟都希望為南派螳螂拳正名：興甯五華沒有周家螳螂拳派，南派螳螂拳應姓朱。他們希望早日將這個誤差告知香港的拳師們。

因為南派螳螂拳一開始是在東江一帶傳承，在揚名之地香港，該拳也被叫做東江螳螂拳，馬九華希望，能將此拳統稱為南派東江螳螂拳，並世代在東江一帶傳承下去。

that he had a great talent for martial arts. Thereafter, he agreed to teach Chen and from 1972 until Ma Ming Sen's passing in 1996 they enjoyed a strong familial teacher-student relationship.

Chen states that Ma Sifu usually taught him from 9pm until 2 or 3 in the morning hours. And that he often would continue to self-train until day break. Some years later, in the vicinity of Luchou town and the Goddess of Mercy Pavilion, Ma Sifu accepted 3 other pupils including Xie Tian Sheng. Today, Chen and Xie continue teaching Chu Gar Mantis in Lao's hometown area.

In 1984, the 77 year old Ma Ming Sen was invited to teach Chu Gar Mantis in nearby Sui Ko Town. There was a large martial arts Association with more than 70 apprentices all by the surname, Yan. Even though Ma taught them, he stated there were very few who really studied.

In 1996, the 90 year old Ma Ming Sen died in his hometown. It is said he stayed up very late until after 5 am, as was his custom, chatting around with all his family as usual, until he said he felt a bit tired and retired. Early the next morning around 6 am, it was discovered he had passed peacefully in his bed.

Ma Ming Sen was the fourth-generation descendant of Chu Gar Mantis in China. He was a disciple of Lao Sui as well as his Son-in-law. Today the Lao and Ma families are still living in the same locations as nearly 100 years before.

Huizhou Disciples go to Meizhou to Research Chu Gar's Patron Deity

Ma Jiuhua Sifu and the others would like to inform all fellow boxers that in China, the legacy of Lao Sui is Chu Gar Mantis and the teaching is descended from ancestor Chu Ya Nan. There is no Chow Gar faction.

In recent years, Southern Mantis has emerged to the public's attention and in the martial arts community many people have known Lao Sui as a great master. Some foreigners have found their way to Lao Sui's hometown to pay respect.

At the same time, the descendants of Chu Gar Mantis in China began a tour to find its deepest roots. In 2008, Ma Jiuhua and over 10 teacher brothers travelled to Hong Kong, Kowloon, and called on the disciples of Lao Sui, including those of Yip Sui and Cheng Wan. However, Ma Jiuhua and all were puzzled that although Lao Sui's Southern Praying Mantis had flourished in Hong Kong as "East River Mantis," it was yet divided into the Chow and Chu factions.

The China descendants of Lao Sui reasoned this error likely occurred because of the Cantonese and Hakka difference in pronunciation. The Chow faction of Lao Sui's disciple, Yip Sui, stated that Zhou Ya Nan was an ancestor of Zhou family village in Xingning; the Chu disciples of Lao Sui in Hong Kong stated that Chu Ya Nan is ancestor.

Chow or Chu family surname
Chow Gar = Chu Gar
Chow = Zhou (Pinyin)
Chu = Zhu (Pinyin)
Gar = Jia (family)
Gao = Jiao (creed)

And so, Ma Jiuhua and the brothers travelled to Meizhou and Xingning, and nowhere could be found a Chow family village or Chow Ya Nan ancestor. However, in Meizhou, Wuhua, Zhuan Shui Zhen, Liantang Village, Chu Ya Nan's identity and boxing was known and identified by the name Chu Gar Gao and Chu Gar Mantis. In China, the Southern Mantis boxing of Wong Fook Go and Lao Sui is Chu Gar Mantis.

Chu Ya Nan is precisely the patron deity of Chu Gar Southern Praying Mantis. In the Ching dynasty, Chu travelled to the Southern Shaolin Temple in Fujian where he followed a Zen monk who had mastered Southern Shaolin boxing. Chu there witnessed a praying mantis eating a bird and from this, in secret, created the boxing that became known as Chu Gar or Chu family, using his own surname, Chu. Later the Zen monk and Chu combined skills.

In order to distinguish between the Northern Mantis boxing, the name of Southern Praying Mantis was attached. Chu Ya Nan later travelled down the East River area to teach to Hakka disciples, and among them was Wong Fook Go, a wandering medicine seller, who taught Lao Sui. (Note: In 2013, Chu Ya Nan's grandson, several generations down the line, still lives in Boluo, nearby Lao Sui's village home.)

In Xingning, from whence 2nd generation, Wong Fook Go, came, 4th generation descendant, elder Fan Jinmao, has written to Ma Jiuhua, to state that in the area where this boxing originated there is only Chu Gar from Chu Ya Nan. There can be found no Chow or Chow Ya Nan. Elder Fan encouraged anyone to come there to investigate for themselves.

And so, today in Lao Sui's village, is a small gallery established by Ma Jiuhua and the others, in honor of Lao Sui's Chu Gar Mantis legacy in China. It is hoped the world over will appreciate Chu Gar Mantis as descended from Chu Ya Nan and passed down five or six generations now. As this boxing school originated along the Guangdong East River, it is the hope of Lao Sui's disciples in China that all may simply refer to it as "East River Southern Praying Mantis." (©今日惠州网，天鹅城网 Excerpted from Dongjiang Times Newspaper ### End)

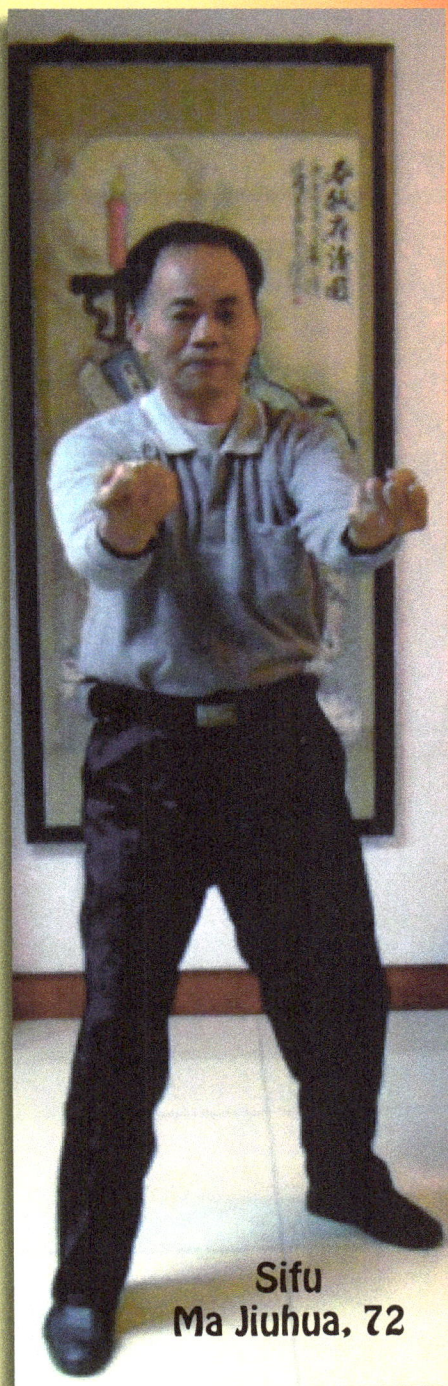

Sifu
Ma Jiuhua, 72

An Interview with Sifu Ma Jiuhua

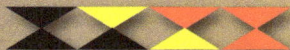

專訪師傅馬九華

馬師傅的父親馬銘
森是一九四五年同
劉水女兒劉秀容結
婚.

Ma Sifu's father,
Ma Mingsen, was
married to Lao
Sui's daughter. The
Ma and Lao family
have been neighbors and relatives for
more than 100 years and remain so today.

When were you, Ma Jiuhua, born? 1942 Where? Hui Yang, Huizhou, neighbors of Lao Sui's family.

Is your family from kungfu? Only my father, Ma Ming Sen, trained Mantis from Lao Sui. Did your grandfathers train kungfu? No, but my grandfather was the same age and a sworn brother of Lao Sui.

Your father, Ma Mingsen, was born in 1907 and passed in 1996 - correct? Yes. Where was he born? He too was born in Hui Yang. After he and grandfather had been in Malaysia, my father, at age 30, went to Hong Kong and learned Mantis from Lao Sui from 1937-1941. After 5 years of training he returned back home in Huiyang, to this very place where we are sitting, by boat on the Dongjiang East River. My father lived with Lao Sui in Hong Kong and taught the classes in the school.

How did you father meet Lao Sui? Our families had long been neighbors in this village. Lao Sui lived from 1879 - 1942 and at age 64 died - correct? Yes. He was about 20 when he started studying Mantis around 1899.

How about Yang Sao? He was a student of Lao Sui in Hong Kong in the early years.

How about Wong Fook Go? Wong Fook Go (Huang Fu Gao) was not a monk but was a vagabond who came from Xingning City when Lao Sui was 20 years old. Wong was a medicine seller and taught what he called Chu Gar Gao. We don't know if he called the Art as Mantis or how old he was when he taught our grandteacher, Lao Sui.

Tell me about your father, Ma Ming Sen's, training of Chu Gar? In 1941, he returned to Huiyang after five years of training in Hong Kong. But, for 30 years did not teach Chu Gar here in the village. Wars and then the Cultural Revolution made it impossible to consider teaching martial art, even illegal to train. In 1962, he trained me, his son, Ma Jiuhua, when I was 20, but times were hard and village life was too poor to concentrate on martial arts. The training consisted of: Chy Sao grinding hands, Duijong two man, Big Hammer fist, Som Bo Gin, and Som Gin Yu Kiu, etc. My father accepted his first student, Chen Jianming, around 1971 or 72.

Your father, Ma Ming Sen, is fourth generation Chu Gar Mantis? Please name the generations? Chu Yan Nan, Wong Fook Go, Lao Sui,

你，馬九華，何時出生？1942在哪裡？惠陽；惠州劉水鄰居的家裡。你的家人以前都會功夫嗎？只是我的父親，馬銘森，跟劉水學朱家螳螂。你的爺爺會功夫嗎？沒有，但我的爺爺和劉水是相同的年齡和劉水結拜的兄弟。

你的父親，馬銘森，出生于 1907 年至 1996 年-過世正確嗎？是。他出生的地方？他出生在惠陽。他和祖父已經在馬來西亞後，我的父親，在年齡 30，去了香港，從 1937年-1941 年學從劉水那裡學朱家螳螂。在 5 年的訓練後他回到家在惠陽區，這個地方是我們住的地方，坐船上東江而回。我父親陪劉水在香港居住，馬銘森代教學生。

那你的父親是如何認識劉水的？我們的家庭長期以來一直在村裡是鄰居關係。劉水從 1879年-1942年和在死亡年齡 64-正確嗎？是。他是約 20水歲時他開始學習螳螂約 1899年。

如何瞭解楊騷？他在早期是劉水在香港的學生。

黃福高怎麼樣?黃福高（黃富 Gao）不是和尚，那是劉水年 20 歲時從興甯市來到一個走江湖。黃是賣藥，教他稱之為朱家教。我們不知道是否他叫朱家螳螂或他多少歲時他那天教我們的 grandteacher，劉水。

告訴我關於你父親的朱家馬銘森培訓嗎？在 1941 年他回到惠陽經過五年的香港方面的培訓。但 30 年沒教朱家螳螂在這村子裡。戰爭，然後文革使得它不可能考慮教學武術，我父親接受了他的第一名學生，陳建明，一九七一年左右。

你的父親，馬銘森，是第四代朱家螳螂嗎？請說出幾代人嗎？朱亞楠、　黃福高，劉水，馬銘森和當前一代是第五。

1984 年，77 歲馬銘森應邀由隋 Ko 深圳惠陽區中的嚴氏族到那裡只有姓嚴才能學朱家螳螂。有 70 多個弟子，但很少真正學習勤奮。

1996 年，90 歲馬銘森死在家鄉嗎？是的 。

Ma Ming Sen, and the current generation is the 5th.

In 1984, the 77 year old Ma Ming Sen was invited by the Yan clan in Sui Ko Zhen district of Huiyang to teach Chu Gar Mantis to only those surnamed Yan. There were more than 70 disciples, but very few who really studied diligently.

In 1996, the 90 year old Ma Ming Sen died in the hometown? Yes, we had a long dinner that evening and everyone sat around chatting until the late hours of the night. Ma Sifu said he was tired and so around 5 am went to lay down. Soon after he was discovered as deceased.

What is the history of Chu Gar? Chu Yan Nan is considered founder and his son, Chu Jin, also taught Mantis. Chu Jin's grandson several generations down the line is still at their home in Boluo, Huizhou today, although, their Mantis was lost a couple of generations before.

Where did Wong Fook Go learn Chu Gar? From the Chu family in Wuhua County. It is estimated Wong Fook Go would be about 160 years old in 2013 and Chu Yan Nan maybe even 200!

One mysterious person, possibly a monk, taught five people. Chu Yan Nam taught Chu Jin who taught Wong Fook Gao. This one mysterious person's five students are responsible for Kwongsai, Chu, and Ox Mantis today. One mysterious person created the art from watching a mantis and a bird fight.

Who were the students of Wong Fook Go besides Lao Sui? We know Wong had other students, but we don't know who or where they are today.

When did Chu Gar Gao become Chu Gar Mantis? And why? Lao Sui called the Art Chu Gar Mantis but we don't know if Wong Fook Go did. Today, some in the Wuhua area still say only Chu Gar Gao. Anecdote: This lends credence to the story that after Lao Sui and Chung Yel Chong's meeting, Chu Gar Gao became Chu Gar Mantis.

From whom did you, Ma Jiuhua learn the Art? How many teachers did you have? I only ever trained with my father, Ma Ming Sen.

Your father lived with Lao Sui for 5 years in Hong Kong and taught many students. How many students did your father, Ma Ming Sen, teach in China? More than 100 students but only ten personal.

朱家教的歷史是什麼？朱亞南被視為創始人和他的兒子朱進也教螳螂。

黃福高除了劉水的學生？ 我不知道還有沒有其他學生。

朱家教什麼時候變得朱家螳螂？ 劉水稱朱家螳螂，但我們不知道是否黃福高說了。今天，五華領域的一些仍然說是朱家教。

誰教了你，我只過跟我的父親學過，馬銘森。

Sifu
Ma Jiuhua
Interview

你父親與劉水5 年在香港教過許多學生。你的父親，馬銘森，在中國有沒有教多少學生？100多名學生。在惠州的多少人？陳建民是我父親的第一學生 。

There were no disciples by ceremony and they called my father as Uncle instead of Sifu. They were all from the same village, very young, and there was no such tradition of ceremony and such. No Sun Toi or ancestral shrine of Mantis, at that time.

How many people in Huizhou? Chen Jianming was my father's first student in 1972 or so and he is still teaching today. Xie Tiansheng is teaching in nearby Boluo and in Zhongsan City, Lin Lunyi is teaching. And in Guangdong Province? Some teach Chu Gar in Wuhua County and that area. Anyone outside Guangdong? That I don't know.

Do you have any foreign students? No Foreign visitors? Yes, mostly from Yip Sui's students. Would you be willing to receive foreign students in the future? Yes! We welcome all to enjoy Chu Gar!

What is your curriculum? Well, I stated the teaching before. There is no shen kung (spirit work) and only staff as a weapon.

How long does it take to teach your students the boxing? There is no formal training, no set curriculum or time.

What are the most important aspects? Mabu (horse), Bridge, Bao Zhuang as guard.

How many hand techniques do you teach?   Maybe about 20. Soft and hard? Ma Ming Sen taught hard strength, no soft strength.

Do you teach weapons? Only staff.

Do you teach qigong? Before the form training included 'bi chi' holding the breath but it is hard to do.

Do you teach Shen gong Spirit work? How long to train this? Lao Sui did train Shen Kung in Huiyang but there is no Shen Kung today.

How about Unicorn dance? How long to teach? No unicorn and no lion today in Lao Sui's hometown.

Anything else about boxing? The history of the Art is Chu - we only say Chu Gar Mantis.

Is the teaching different in each of the 5 areas; Xingning, Wuhua, Meixian, Shantou, Meizhou? Some say only Chu Gar Gao not Mantis. Some have combined Sombogin into other forms and their form names are different. Some have high horse, some have long (low) horse.

59

任何現存有劉水的書嗎？ 沒有只有詩歌（在牆上的兩個頁）。

Sifu
Ma Jiuhua
Interview

福建白鶴、 龍心、白眉 等任何與朱家連接有什麼關係嗎？林耀桂（龍）、 李義（李家）、張禮泉（白眉i）和劉水全部來自這同一個地方、 惠陽。

我朱家師傅，鄭運， 他的祖籍也是惠陽區。他經常訪問你嗎？有他陪你的師母一起過來幾次。

So we know of High horse, Low horse, and Maoshan Chu Gar? 36/72/108? I did not see the Maoshan Chu Gar. There is some 'mak' point training including seasonal points but no 108 form.

Any books extant from Lao Sui? No, only the poetry (two pages on the wall - page 156).

What about Chow Gar? Yip Sui (Ip Shui)? In China, we only know Chu Gar. The teaching of the Chu family and Wong Fook Go came to Lao Sui and us, from the Wuhua area. Anyone is welcome to visit for themselves to inquire about this.

What about Kwongsai Mantis / Iron Ox Mantis / Chung Yel Chong / Lam Sang? We don't know about them - We only know one mysterious person taught five and that it spread into three branches.

Any Connection to Fujian Crane, Dragon, Bak Mei, etc? Lam Yu Kwei (Dragon), Chueng Li Chuen (Bak Mei), and Lao Sui were all from this same place, Huiyang, and perhaps spent time together drinking tea.

My Chu Gar Sifu, Cheng Wan, was from here in Huiyang. Did he visit you often? Some times with your Simu, his wife.

Lao Sui was 20 years old when he studied Mantis and at 24 left his Master Wong in Huiyang and travelled to Hong Kong to teach. That was 1899 - 1903 when he studied Mantis and around 1904 he went to Hong Kong. But it is said he didn't start teaching in Hong Kong until some years later, like 1915 - 1937? This isn't clear.

Wong Fook Go - how old was he when teaching Lao? Possibly 60 -70 years old. Chu Ya Nan was how old when teaching Wong Fook Go? We can't be sure.

Is Lao Sui's son still living? No.

Did Lao Fu Yuan, Lao Sui's brother have Mantis students? No. He passed in the 1970s but his son, Xiang Nan, who you met, is 95 and still lives in the old house Lao Sui built in 1936. Xiang Nan did study with his uncle Lao Sui in Hong Kong after training medicine in Shanghai, in the 1930s.

There is a exhibition gallery of Mantis in Hong Yuen village today, where? In my old home, next door to Lao's. Just a small room with photographs around the wall, and many recent pictures.

End

劉水20 歲時他學習螳螂和 24歲 在惠陽離開他黃師傅，前往香港
教。那就是當他學習了螳螂 1899年-1903 年和約 1904 他去了香
港。但它說他沒教 1915年-1937 年開始直到幾年後，在香港教學
嗎？這還不清楚。

黃福高他多少歲時教劉水嗎？可能 60-70 歲。朱亞南是多少歲教黃
福高嗎？我們不能肯定。

劉水兒子仍然在嗎？他已經去世了。

Liu Fu Yuan，劉水的兄弟有螳螂學生嗎？沒有他大概在 一九七幾年
去世，可是你見過他的兒子劉湘南 95歲，仍然生活在劉水建于 1936
年的老房子。劉 湘南一九三幾 年代在上海學醫學研究後來去香港跟
他的伯父劉水學朱家螳螂。

今天，在香園村有螳螂展覽畫廊的地方嗎？在我的老家，在劉水的隔
壁。只是一小間房周圍的牆上，很多最新圖片照片。

＃ ＃ ＃ 結束

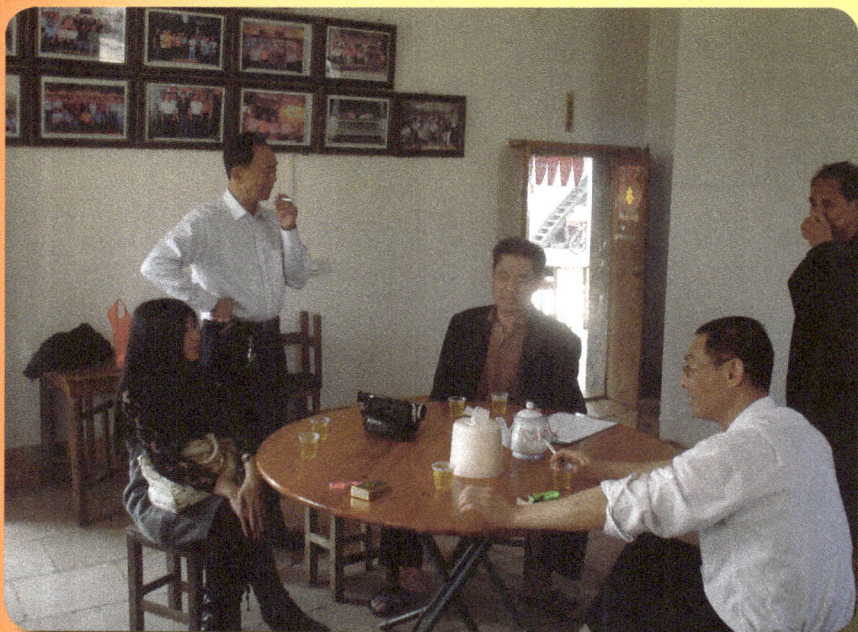

The Mantis Exhibition Gallery at Lao Sui's Village home today is a
small room displaying photographs, many recent.

Chu Gar Mantis
Principles and Fundamentals

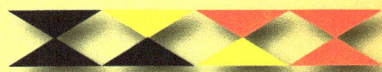

基本功

Oral Song
Horse
Hand Skills
Form Training

Huizhou Southern Praying Mantis Boxing
惠州南螳螂武術協會
Chen Jian Ming Association
陳建明 師傅

Chen Jian Ming is the first student of Ma Mingsen and began training in 1972. Today, he carries forward Chu Gar Mantis and has appeared in local newspapers and television promoting the legacy of Lao Sui's Chu Gar Mantis in Huizhou, Lao Sui's hometown.

The above plaque details his School:

Creed: Respect your parents, respect your mentors, respect their guidance; learn benevolence, learn righteousness, learn kung fu.

Posture: Stance not Chinese character 8 or ding but both, sink the shoulder, drop the elbow, swallow the chest, hunch the back.

Tactics: Strike from the heart; you do not strike, I do not start; qinna - seize and grasp; cross via a bridge; no bridge then create one; advance the bridge preceded by hand.

包椿

The following
pages detail
basic skills
in Chu Gar Mantis
基本功

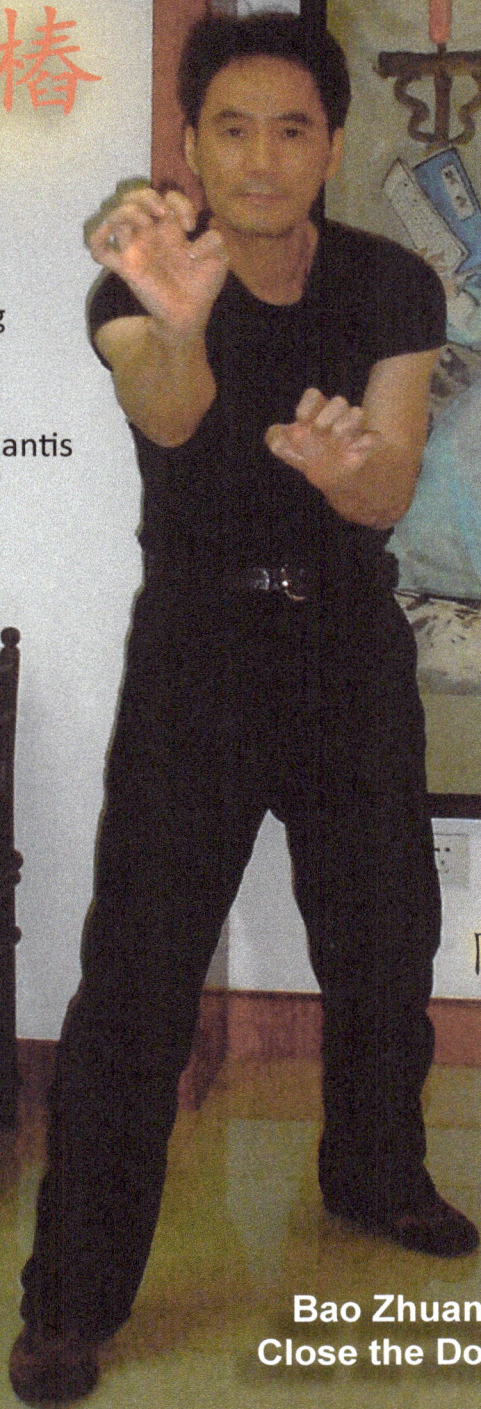

師傅
陳建明

**Bao Zhuang
Close the Doors**

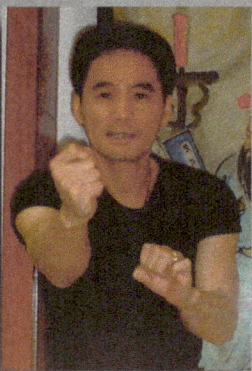

絞槌

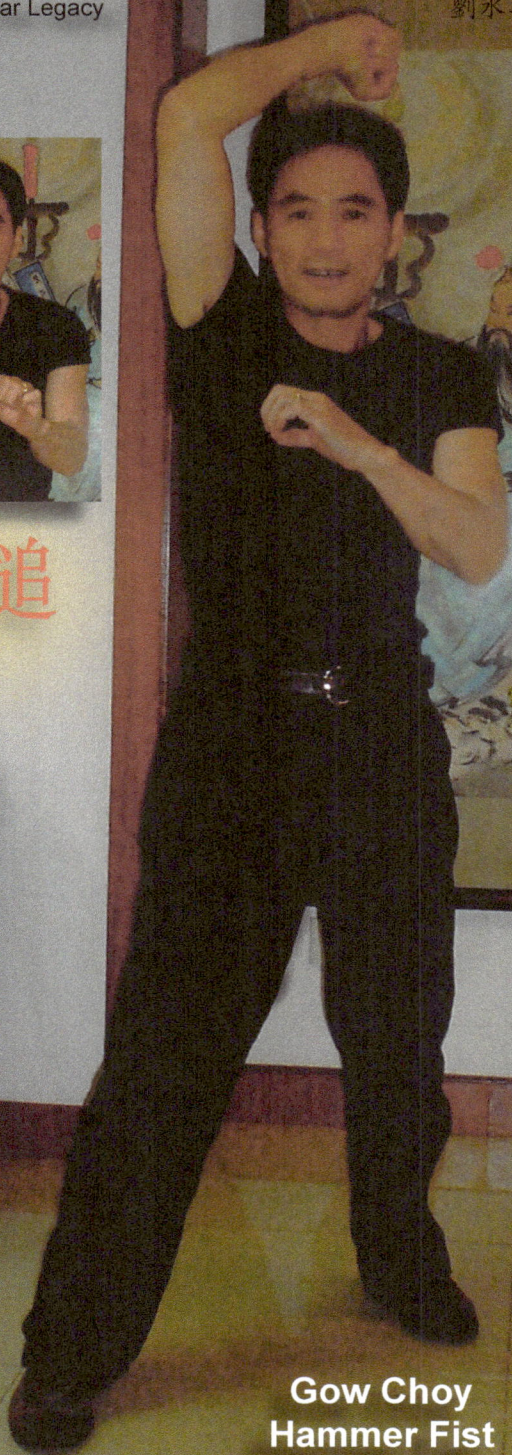

**Gow Choy
Hammer Fist**

搖手

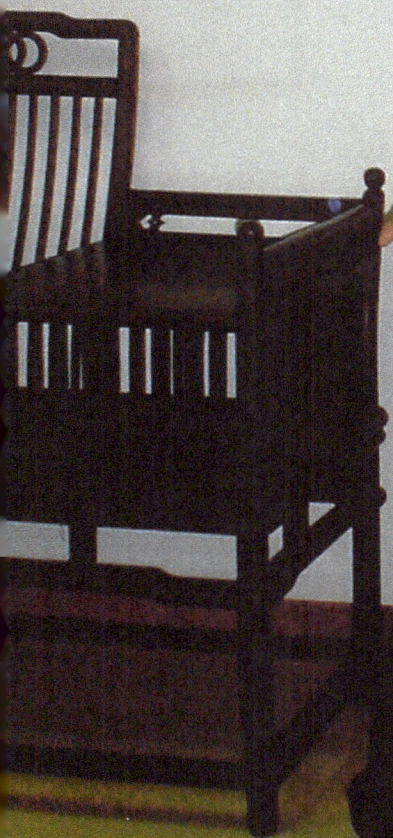

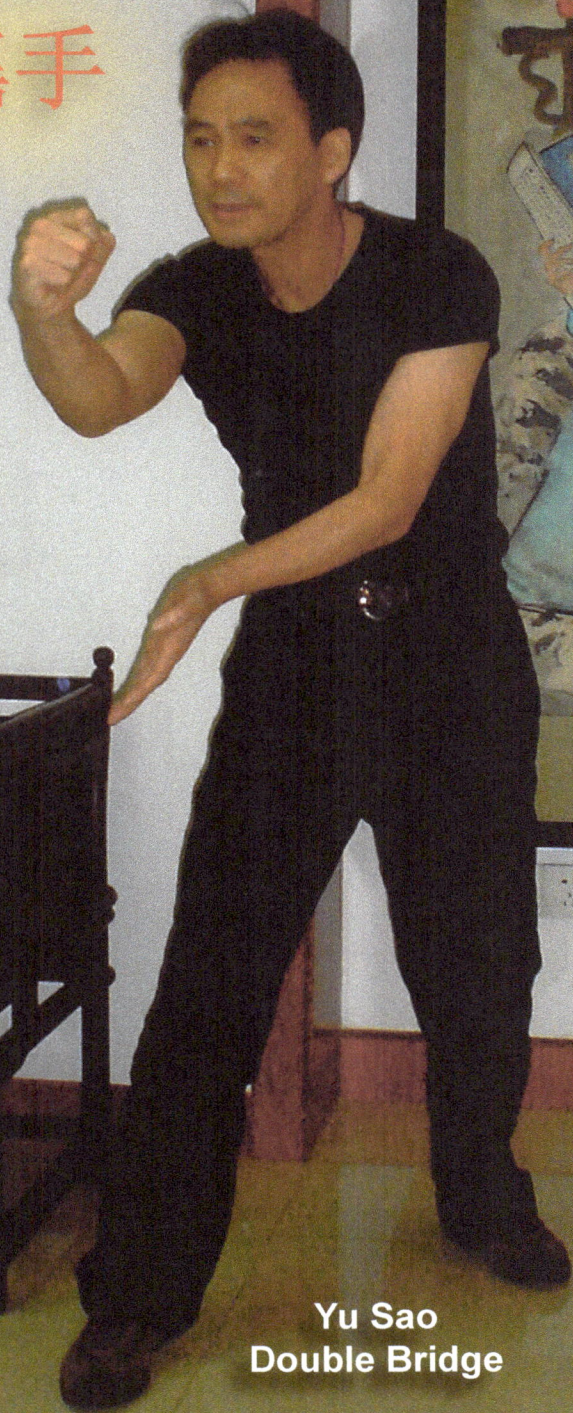

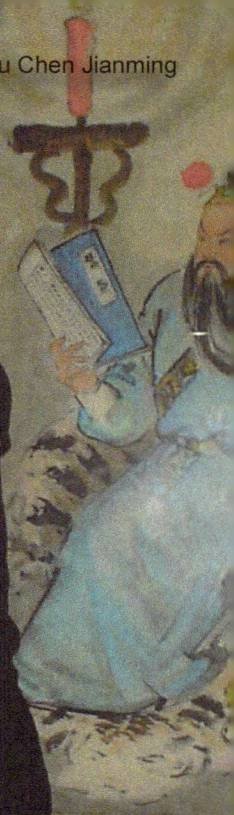

**Yu Sao
Double Bridge**

傳手

**Chuan Sao
Right**

傳手

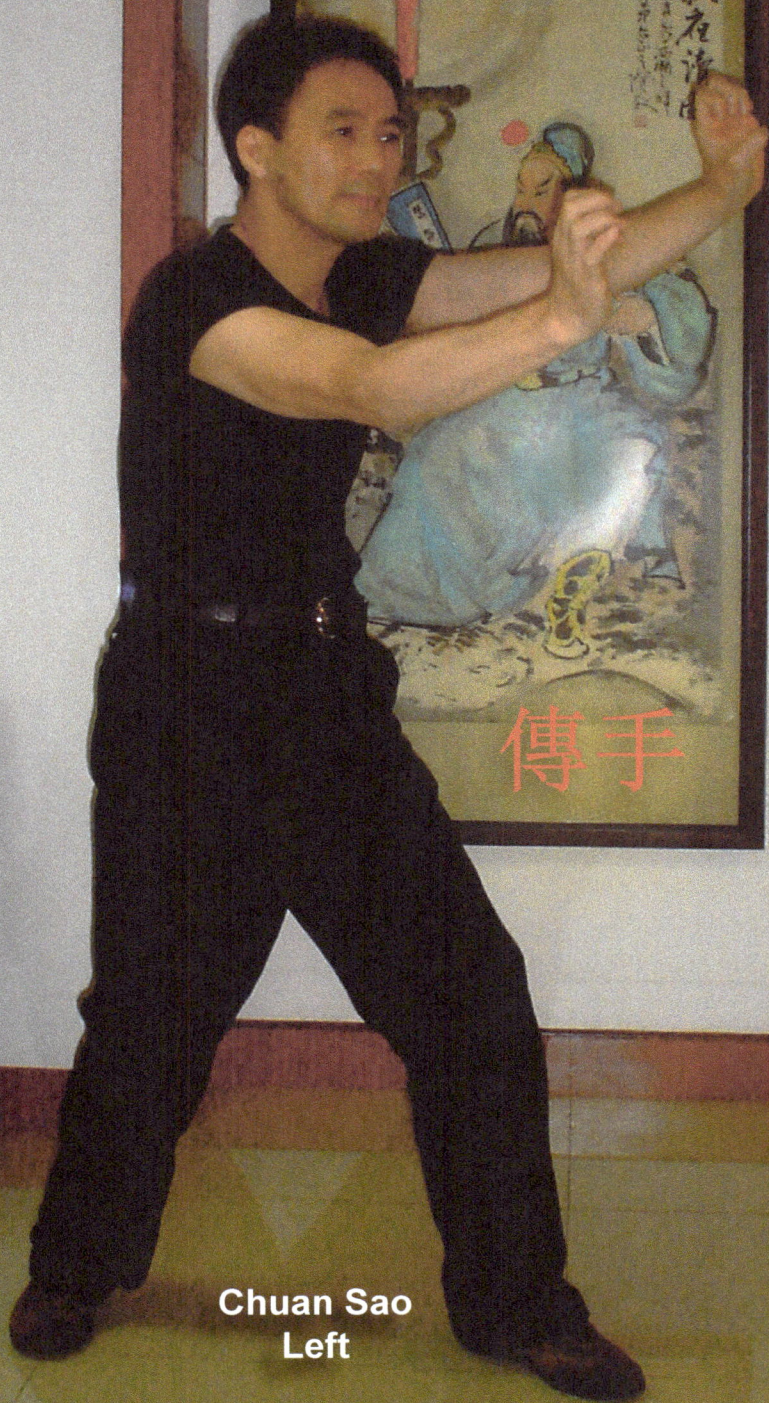

**Chuan Sao
Left**

捯手

鄒水功夫遺產在中國

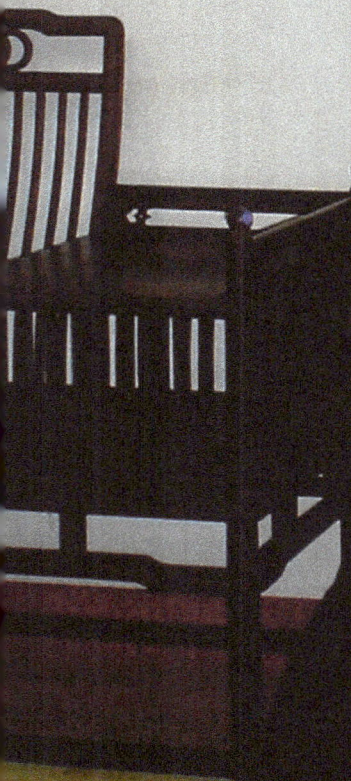

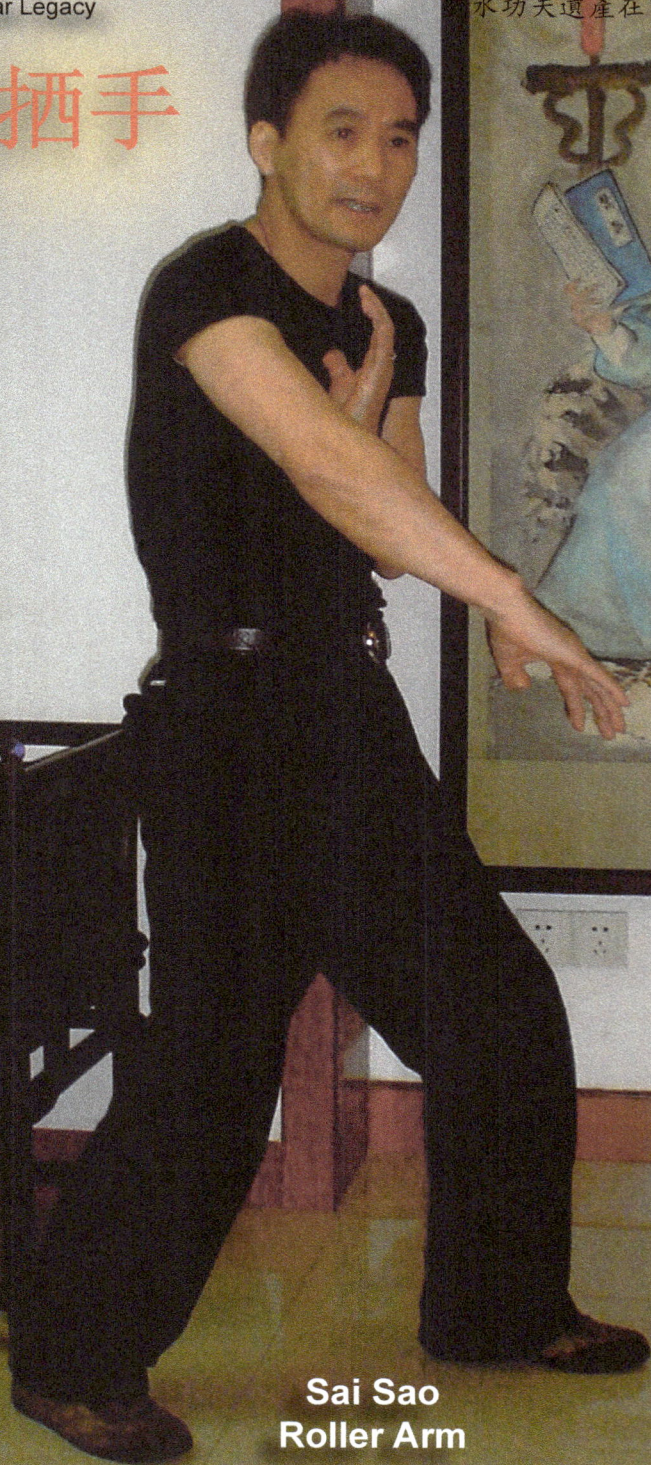

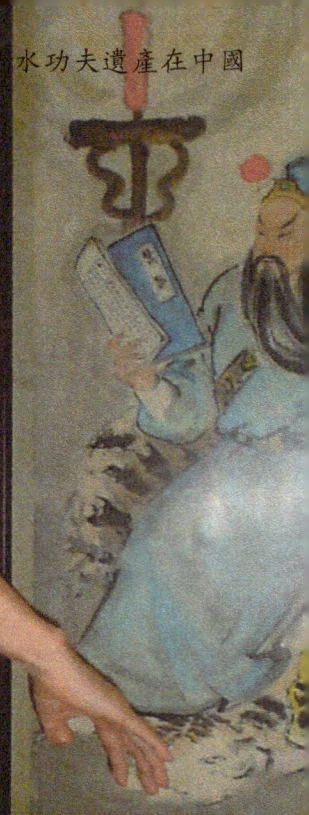

Sai Sao
Roller Arm

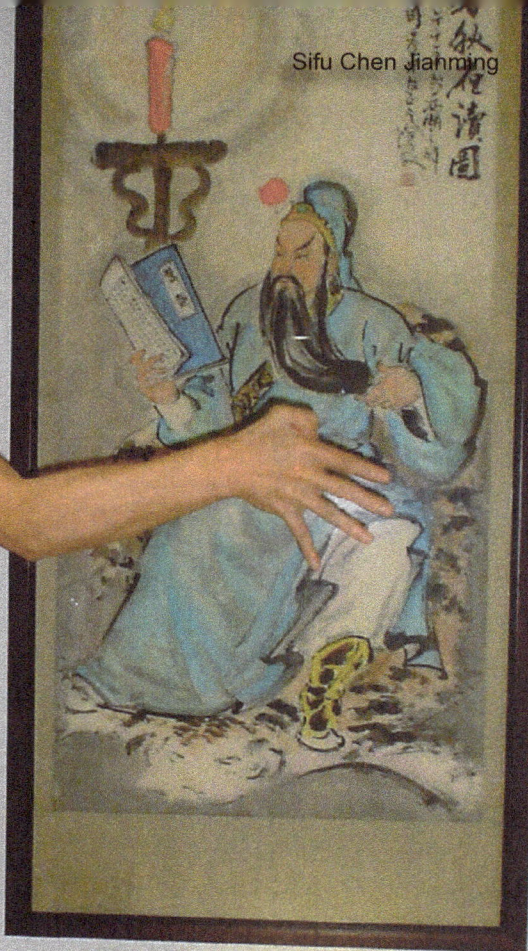

押手

Ya Sao
Lock Hands

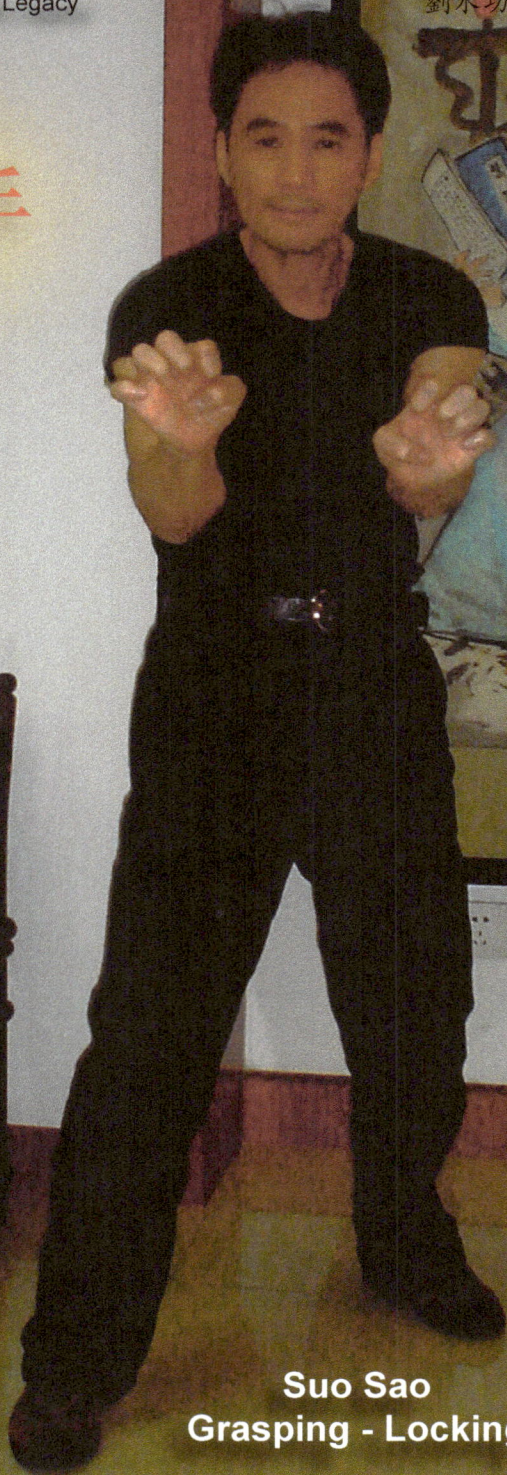

鎖手

Suo Sao
Grasping - Locking

抖手

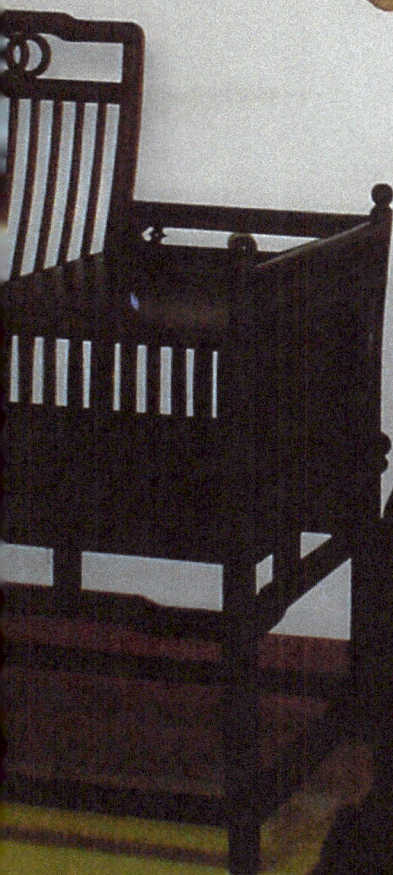

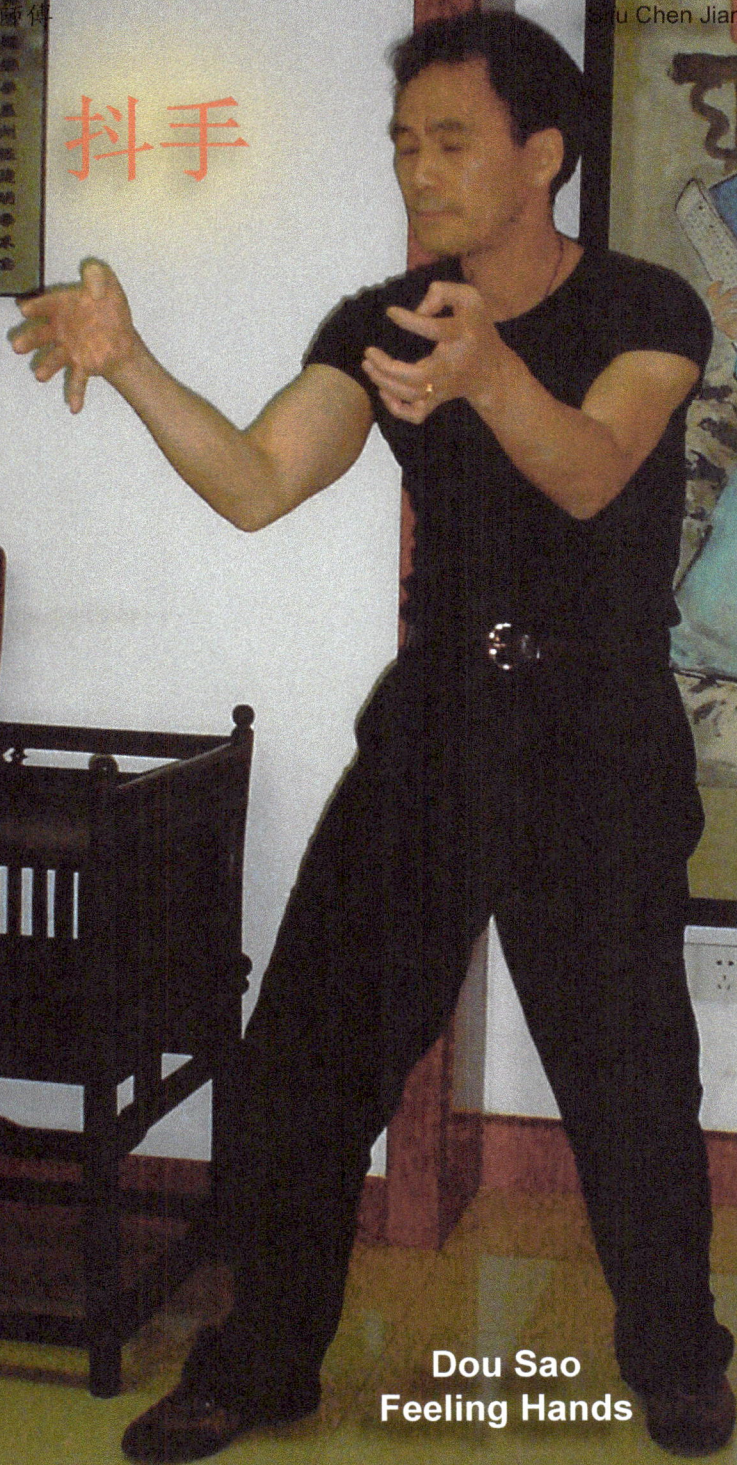

Dou Sao
Feeling Hands

73

劉水功夫遺產在中國

割手

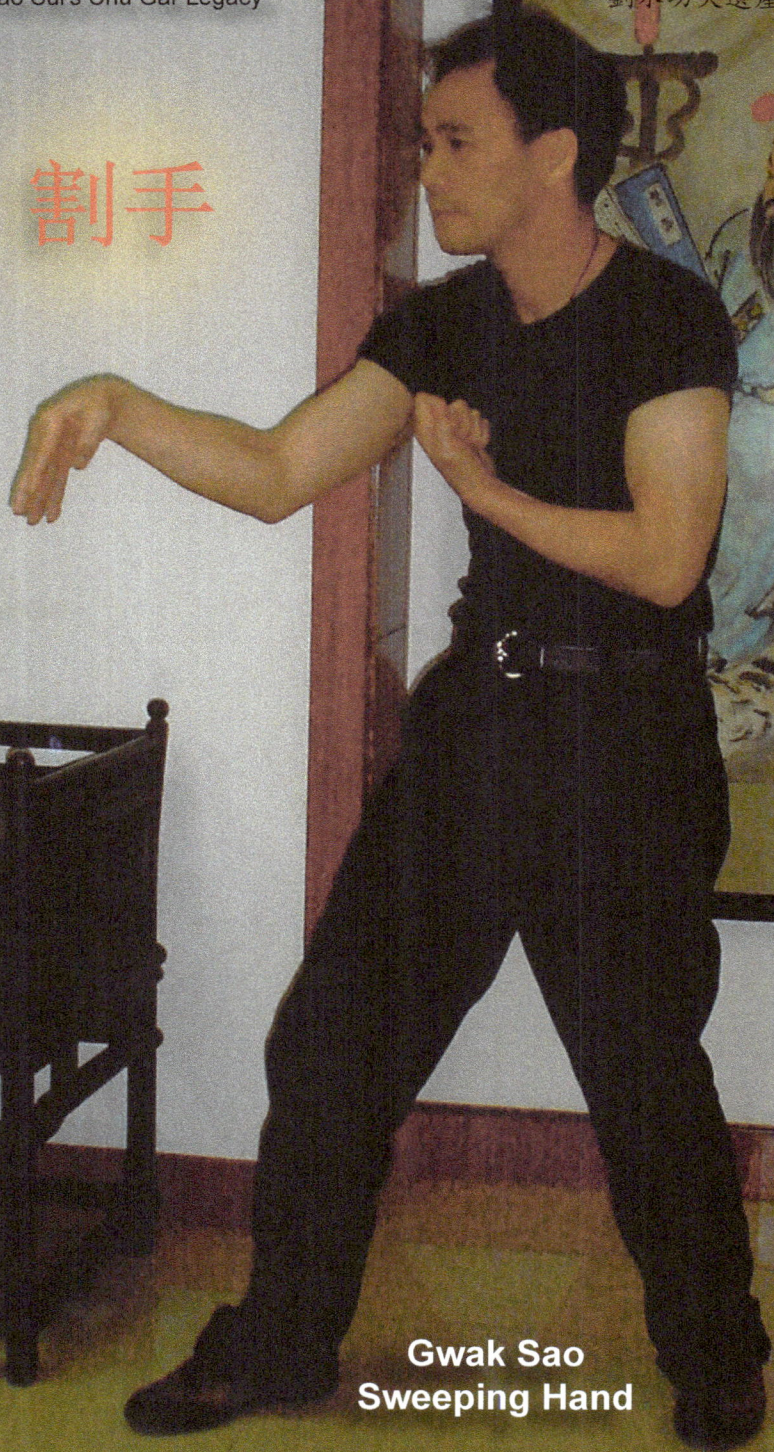

**Gwak Sao
Sweeping Hand**

批手

**Pi Sao
Feeling Hands**

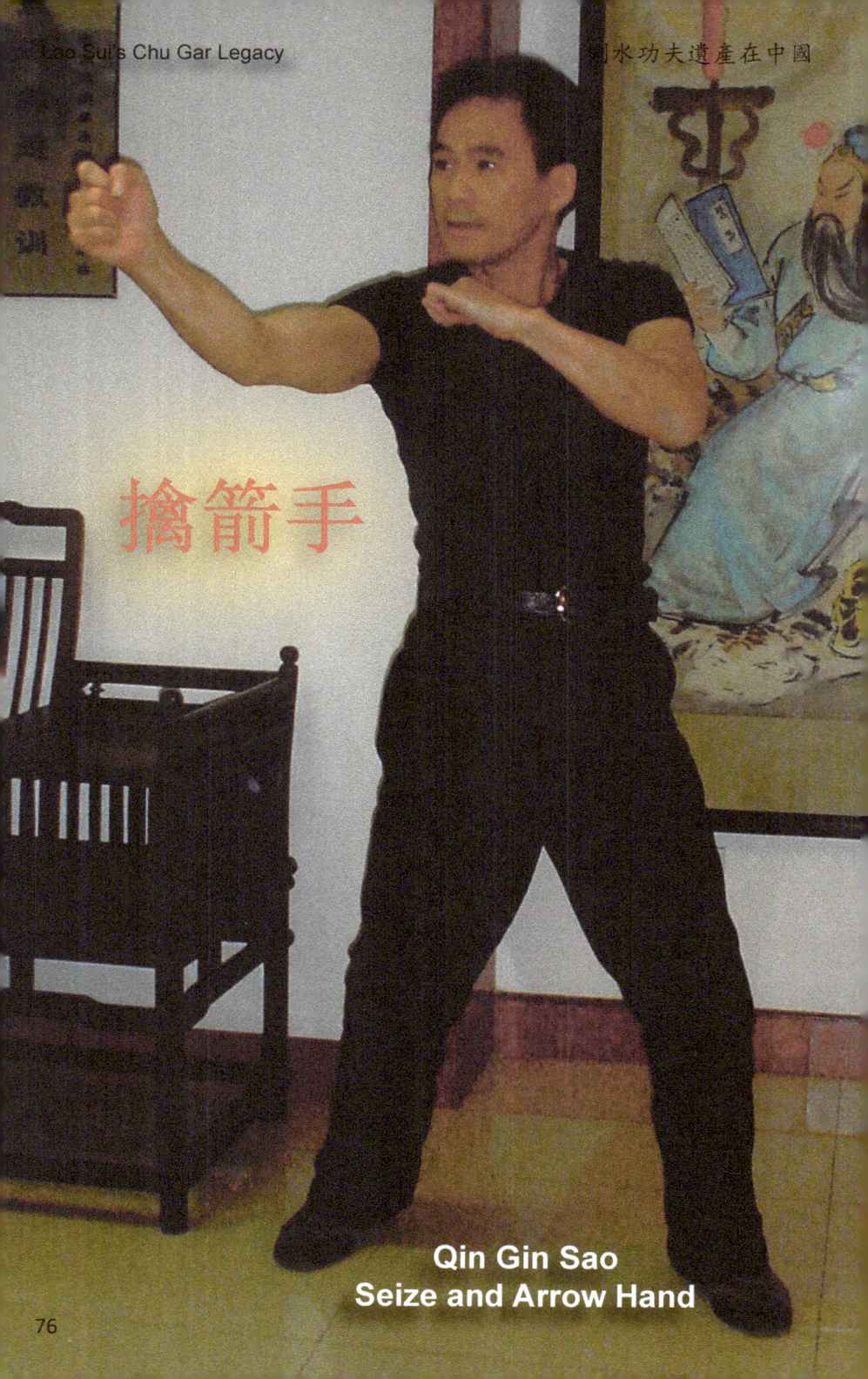

擒箭手

**Qin Gin Sao
Seize and Arrow Hand**

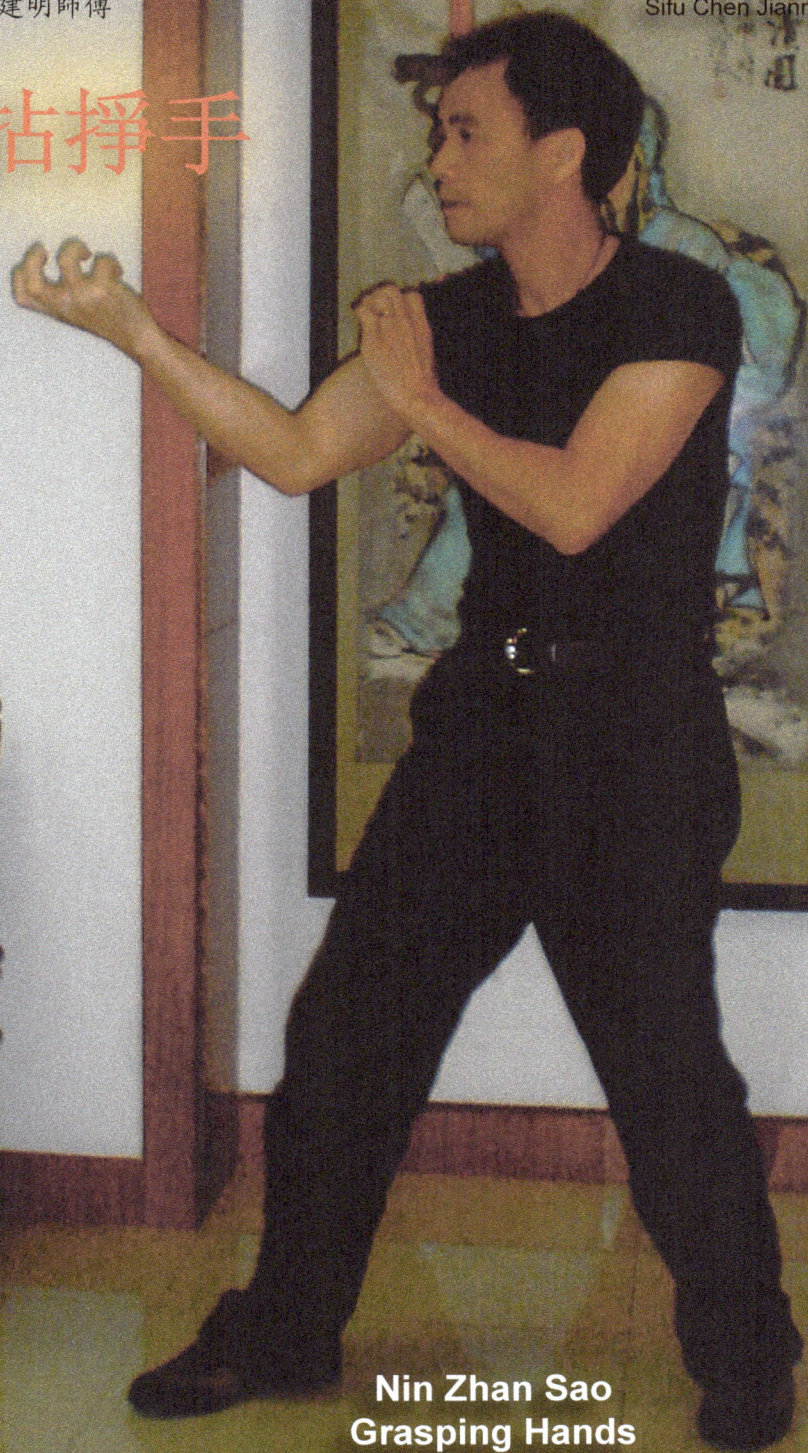

拈掙手

Nin Zhan Sao
Grasping Hands

Form

Training single man forms and shadowboxing is to know one's self. Sticky hand and two man training is to know others.

Som Bo Gin 三步箭
Som Gin Yu Kiu 三箭搖橋

I offer this form pictorial as a record only. It is impossible to teach form correctly by a book, but, the pictorial will serve as a reminder of the sequence. It is always best to seek a competent teacher. Step by step DVD instruction is a good second choice and also useful.

If you do not understand the principles and fully train the two man fundamental skills first, then **form training** is a house without a foundation; a house built upon sand.

Your Mantis house is empty without becoming skillful at the fundamental two man footwork, two man hand skills, sticky hand and two man forms. Once these are correct, your single man form will be correct. Shadowboxing alone will lead to failure in self-defense.

Having said that, the beginning of training is by self-study alone. You must ingrain the Mantis body posture and internal work and that can only be accomplished by oneself. Form is an essential self-study tool.

Important elements to remember:
* 18 points of internal training
* Natural breathing, holding the breath
* Stepping pattern
* Relaxed strength not tense and stiff
* Float, sink, swallow, spit
* Offensive-Defensive
* Three Power Gin - arrow, forward, scissors
* Warrior Intent

The following pages show step by step the primary postures, in sequence, of the first two Chu Gar forms, Som Bo Gin, and Som Gin Yu Kiu. Training from this book alone, you may first stand and hold each posture for 3-5 minutes. When you remember the sequence without fail, then you may link the postures together in "form" by movement. Seek a competent instructor or follow a DVD.

套路

個人套路練習和擬敵
單練是要學生認識自
我雙人黐手和對拆培
養學生瞭解對手

三步箭和三箭搖橋

我只收錄兩個套路做為範例, 學習武術僅依賴書中平面圖片是幾乎不可能的事, 連續圖解僅能幫助 你記憶套路的正確順序, 但無法取代稱職的老師, 退而求其次, 循序漸進淺入深的教學光碟也是一個選擇。

如果你不瞭解基本原則, 熟悉雙人對練, 套路的訓練將猶如建餘流沙上的房子。

沒有基本的步法, 沒有雙人對練, 沒有黐手的訓練, 你的房子將是空蕩蕩, 套路的訓練也只是徒然, 擬敵單練也無法達到防身的初衷。
螳螂拳的訓練從認識感受自我開始, 你必須掌握並遵循螳螂拳的正確姿勢和內在運作原則, 套路練習就是綜合上述原則的訓練。

必須牢記重點:
- 十八點內在訓練
- 自然呼吸, 屏住呼吸
- 走馬
- 鬆而不軟, 勁而不僵
- 浮, 沉, 吞, 吐
- 攻擊和防守
- 三勁 – 發勁如箭嗾, 直線穿透, 剪力
- 求勝意志

學習朱家螳螂拳的三步箭和三箭搖橋, 可依下列連續圖解, 練習每式的定式三到五分鐘, 再將定式串成套路練習, 練習時最好有老師指正或教學光碟參考

Three Step

Step

三步箭

Arrow

Boxing

Chu Gar Mantis
Shadowboxing Forms

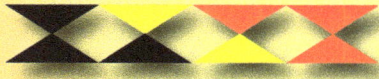

The following pages are a pictorial of the Three Step Arrow
boxing form as played in Lao Sui's Village today.

(Refer to the
Southern Mantis Press book, "Som Bo Gin Two Man Form,"
for the meaning of Som Bo Gin.)

謝添勝師傅
三步箭拳演示（劉水故居）

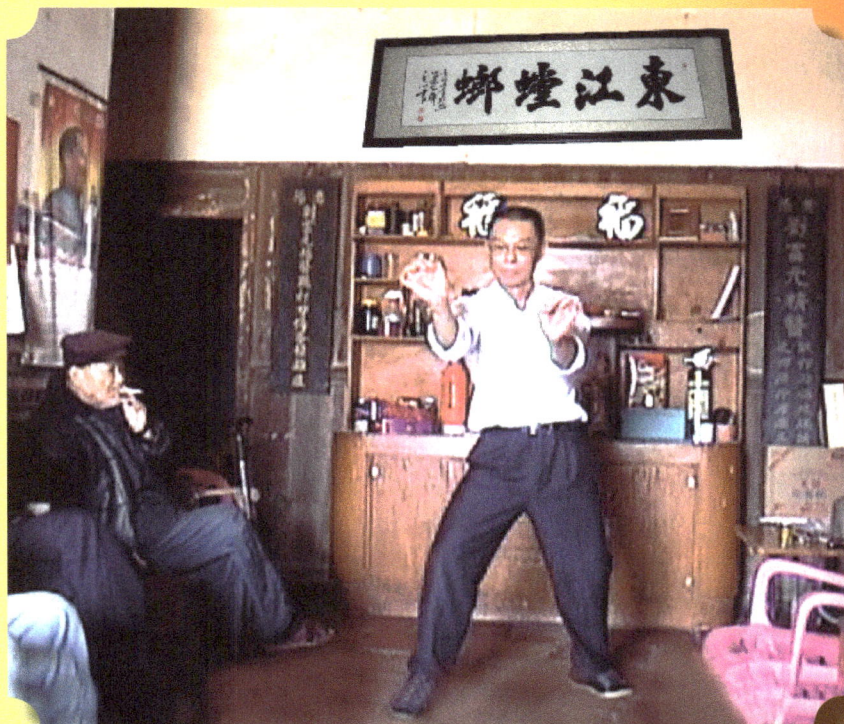

Above: Sifu Xie Tiansheng plays Som Bo Gin shadowboxing in Lao Sui's 1936 home as Lao Xiang Nan, 95, looks on in 2013. Lao Xiang Nan, smoking a cigarette, is Lao Sui's nephew and the oldest relative of Lao Sui today. He trained Mantis with Lao Sui in the 1930s in Hong Kong. The placard above the mantle states Dongjiang East River Praying Mantis.

上文： 謝添勝師傅在劉水1936年故居演示三步箭，旁坐吸煙者為劉水家族高齡九十五歲的 劉湘南先生，為劉水現存最老的學生 。 他在1930年在香港與劉水學藝。牆上的橫匾寫的是東江螳螂。

Xie Tiansheng Sifu is one the early students of Ma Mingsen in the home village and began training in 1980 in the Guan Yin Temple Town.

謝添勝是馬銘森師傅在香園村早期的學生， 開始於1980年在觀音閣鎮。

THREE STEP ARROW BOXING

Opening
Salute
With
Right
Phoenix
Eye

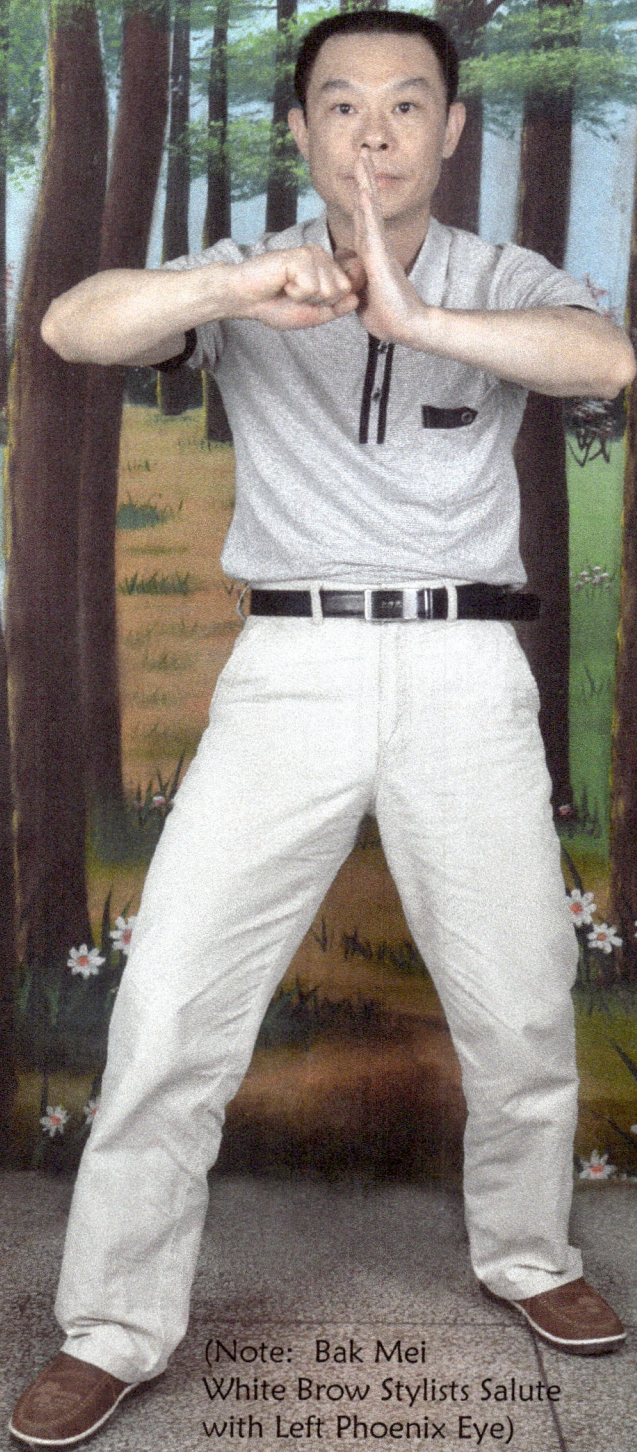

1

Opening
salute
right
horse

82

(Note: Bak Mei
White Brow Stylists Salute
with Left Phoenix Eye)

谢添胜師傅

三步箭

2

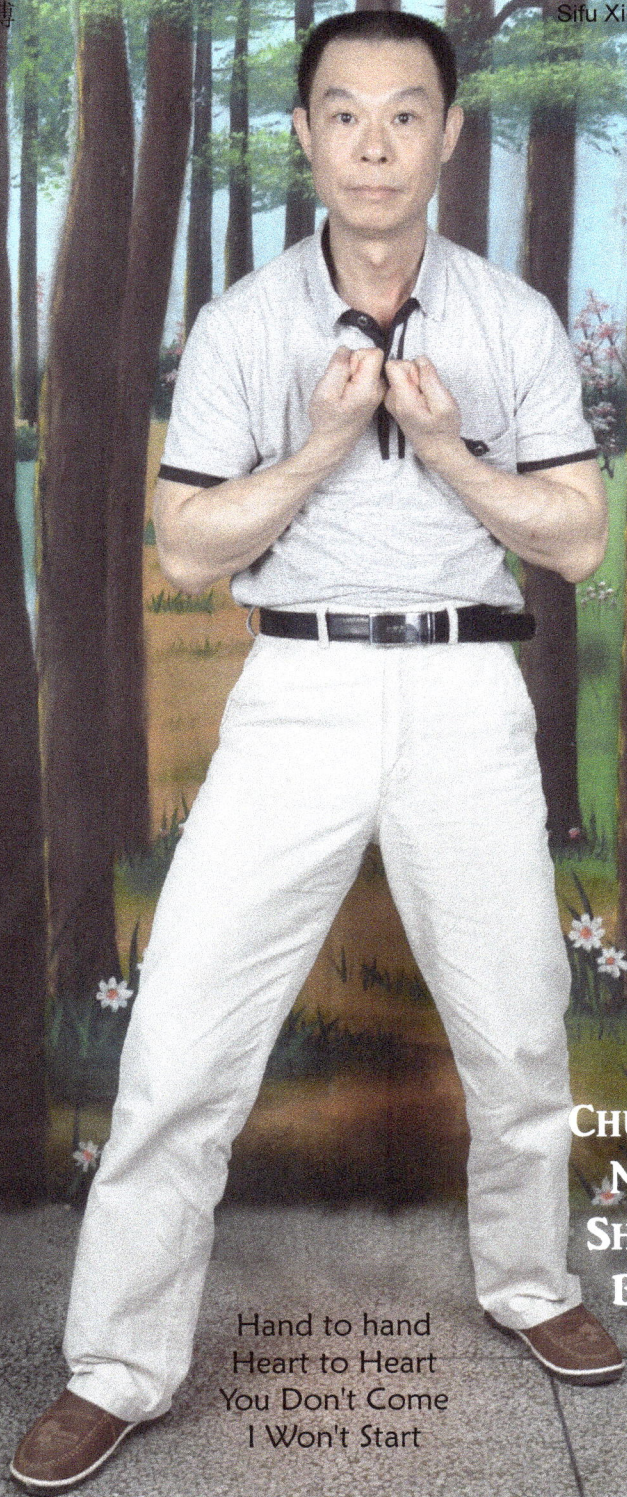

CHU GAR MANTIS SHADOW BOXING

Hand to hand
Heart to Heart
You Don't Come
I Won't Start

THREE
STEP
ARROW
BOXING

Opening
Sequence
Includes
Postures
#1 - #11

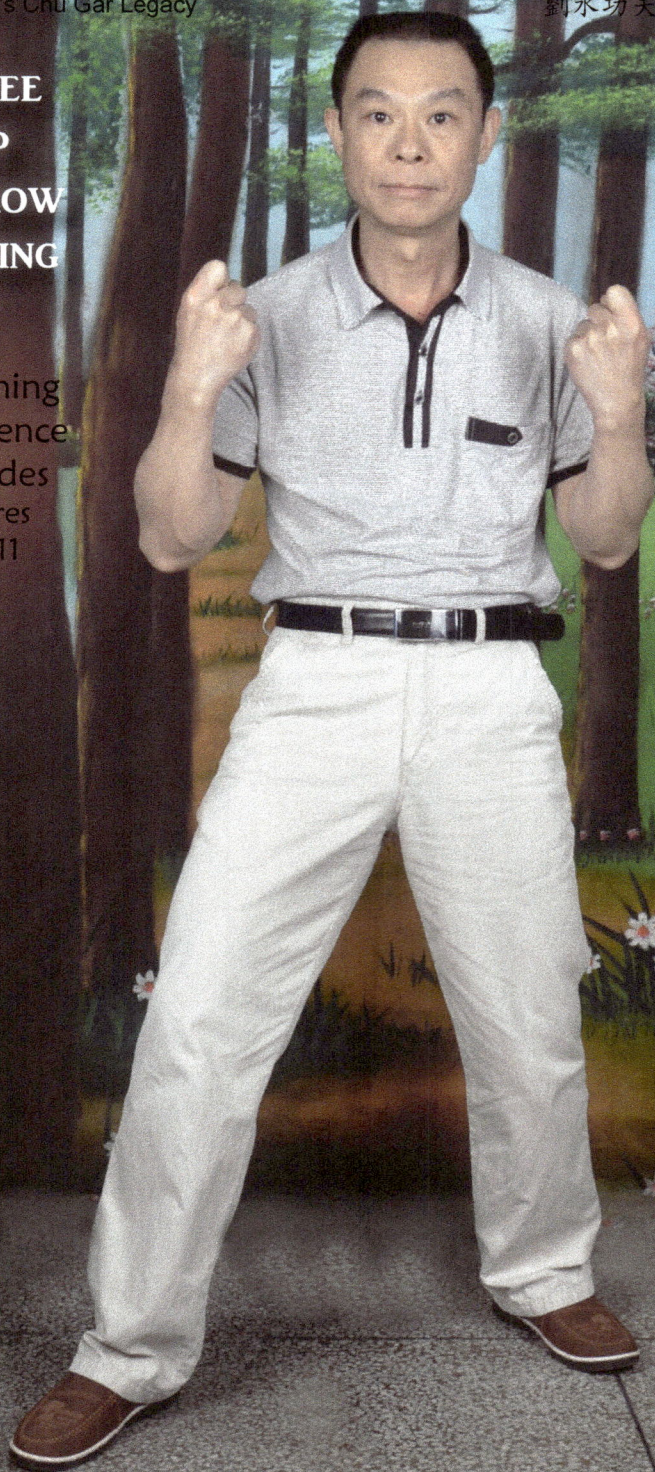

3

三步箭

4

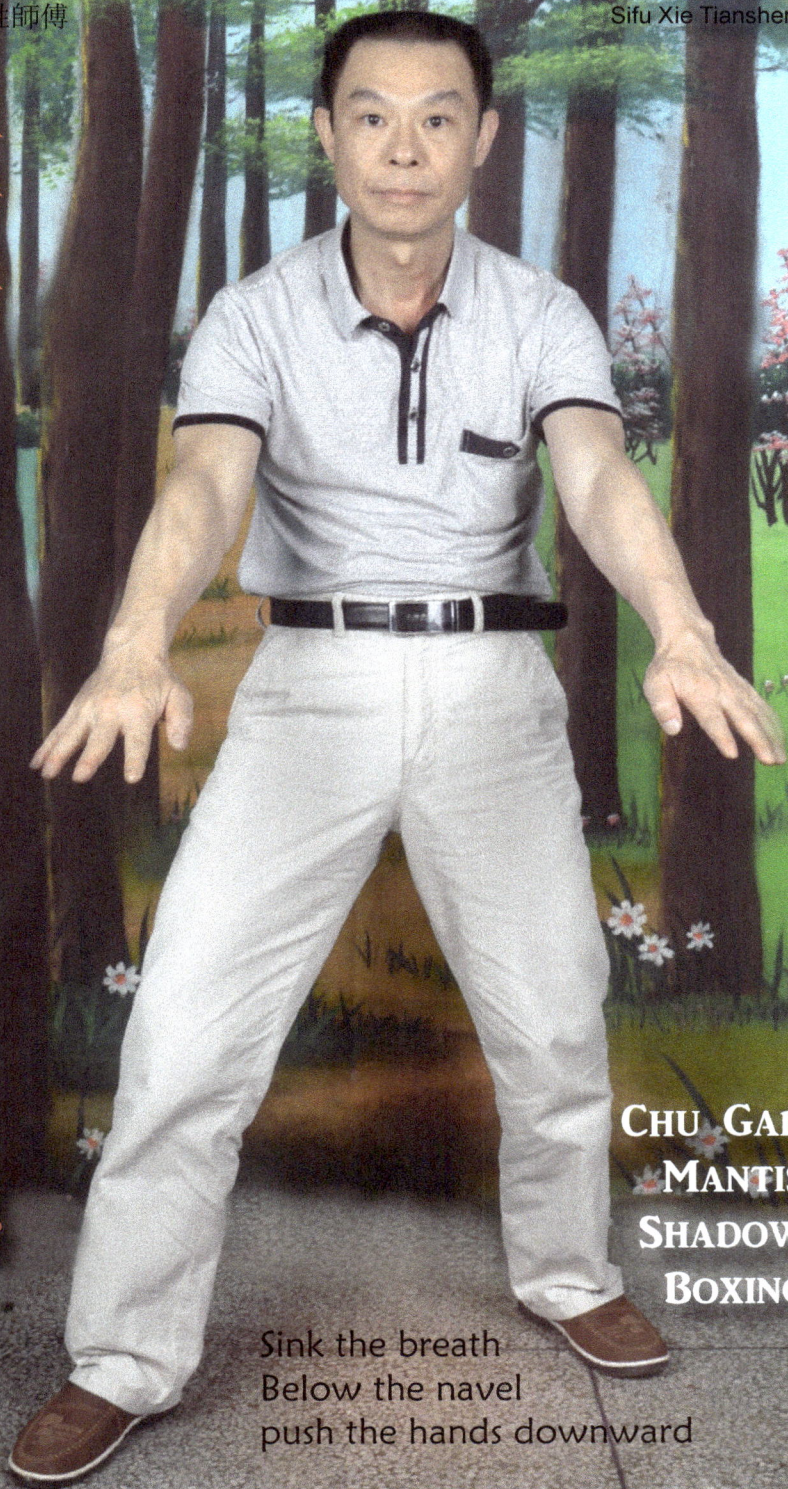

CHU GAR
MANTIS
SHADOW
BOXING

Sink the breath
Below the navel
push the hands downward

THREE STEP ARROW BOXING

5

The movements of the Opening Sequence develop rib and spring power used for explosive force

三步箭

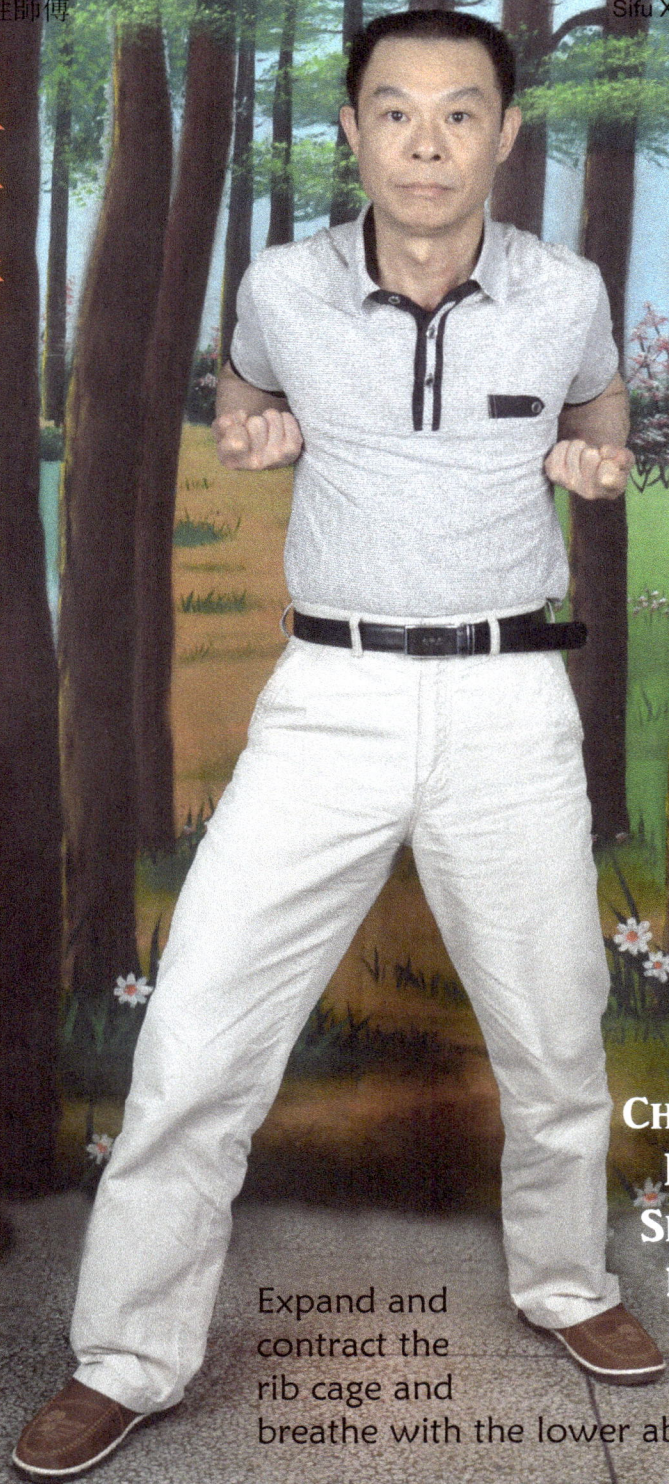

6

CHU GAR
MANTIS
SHADOW
BOXING

Expand and
contract the
rib cage and
breathe with the lower abdomen

THREE
STEP
ARROW
BOXING

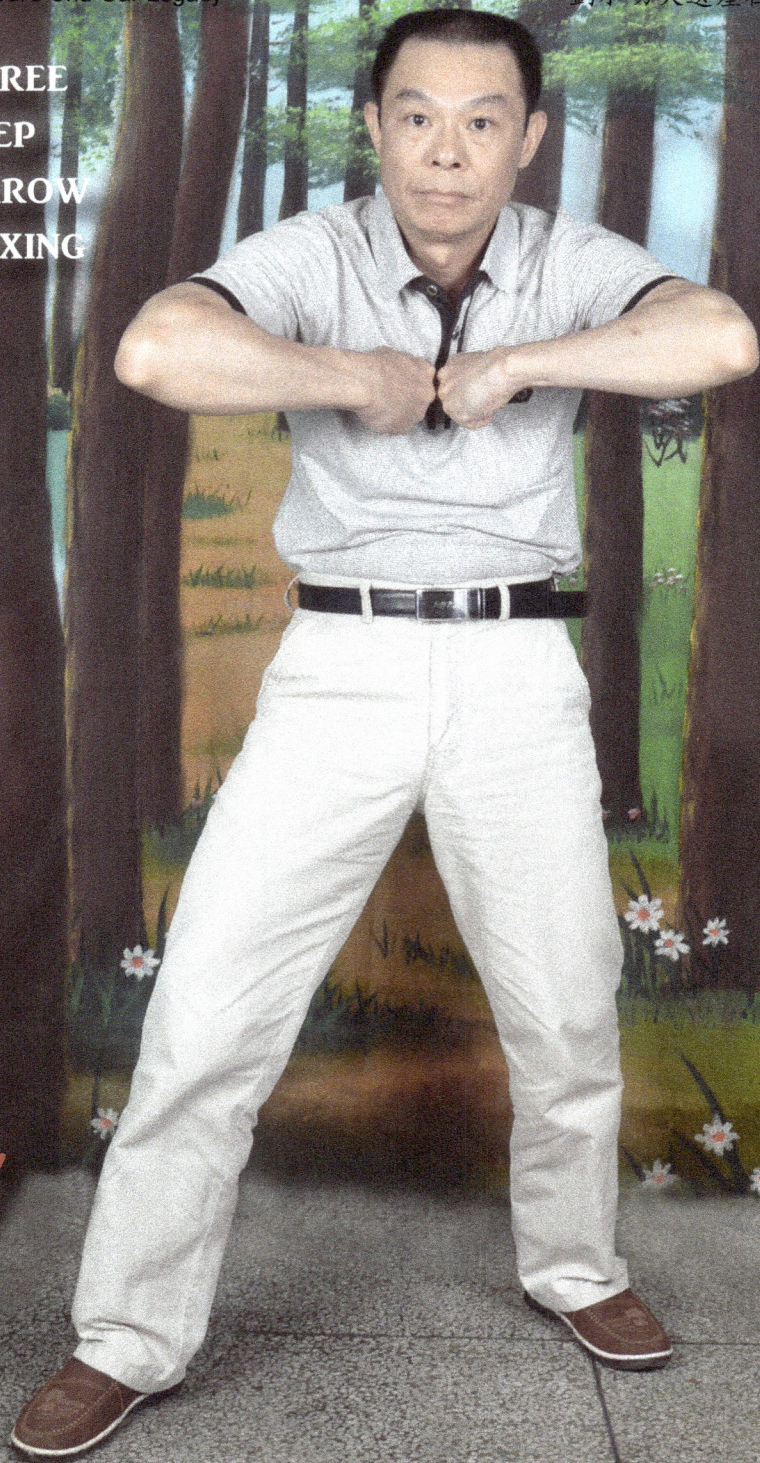

7

三步箭

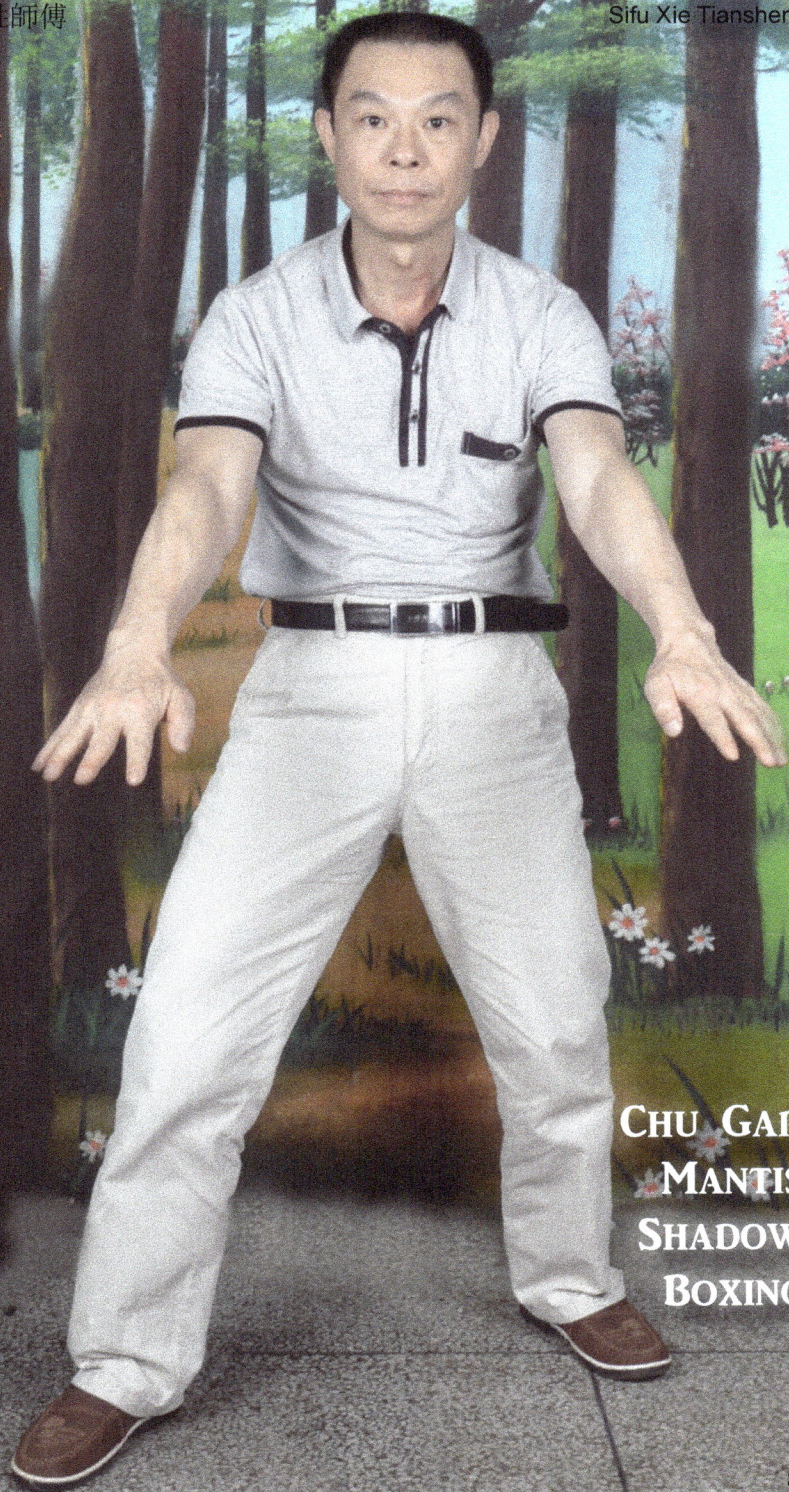

8

CHU GAR
MANTIS
SHADOW
BOXING

THREE
STEP
ARROW
BOXING

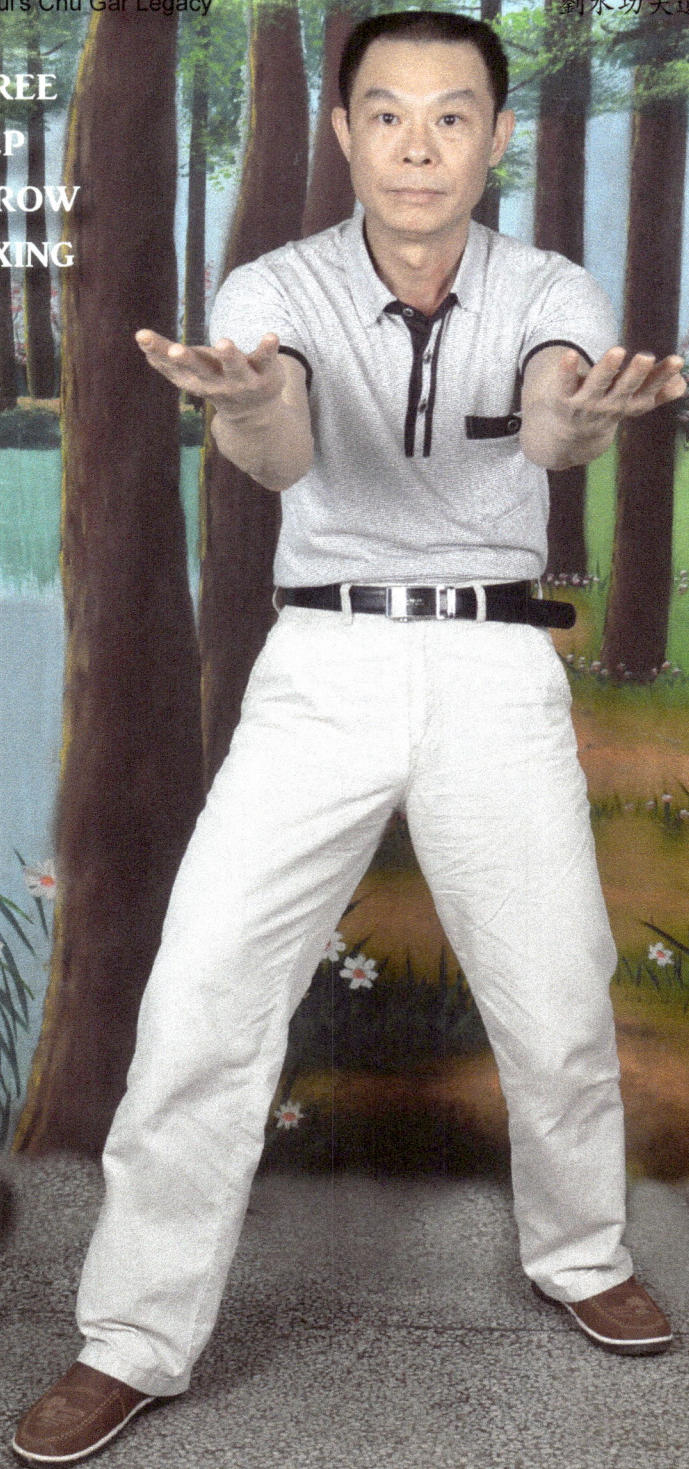

9

三步箭

10

**CHU GAR
MANTIS
SHADOW
BOXING**

Quickly turn the
palms over and spear the fingers
outward stretching from the shoulder

THREE
STEP
ARROW
BOXING

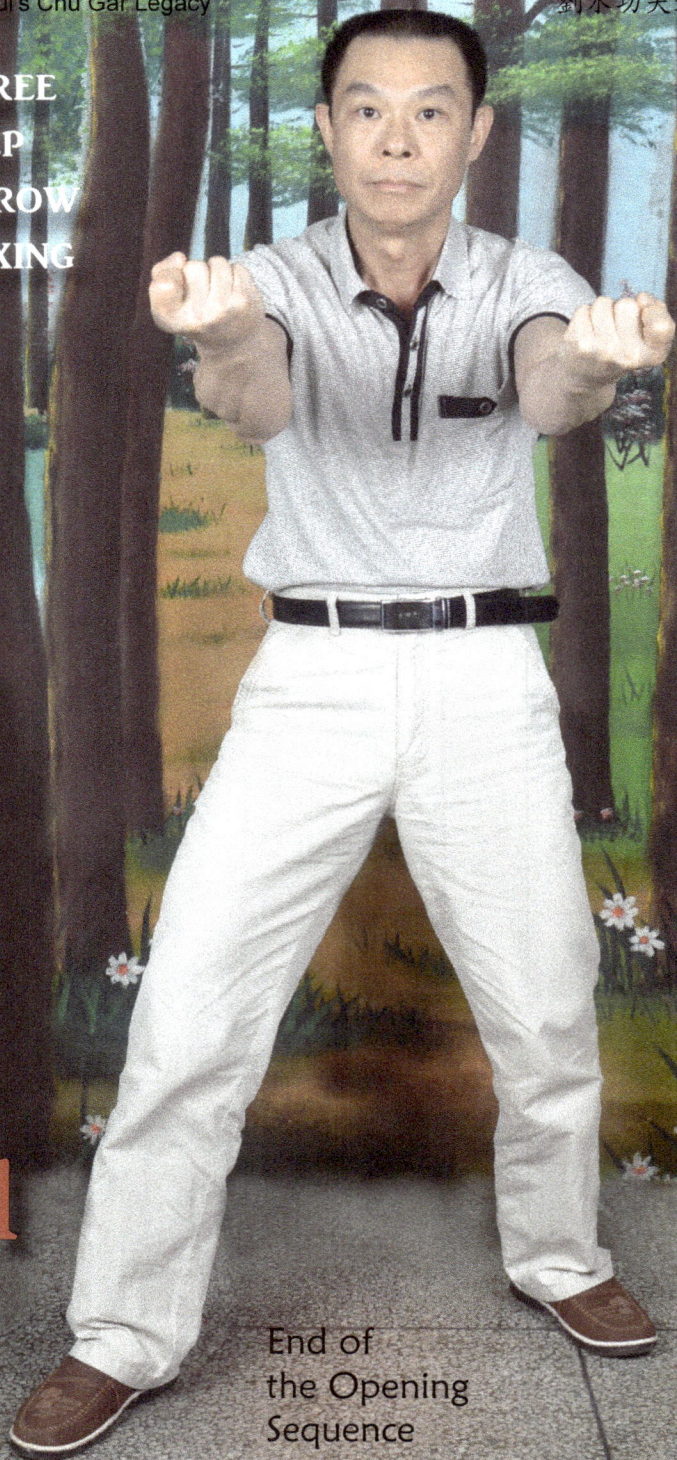

11

End of
the Opening
Sequence

Sifu Xie Tiansheng

三步箭

Double Bridge
Phoenix Eye
strikes
are followed
by Bil Jee
Exploding
Finger
strikes

**CHU GAR
MANTIS
SHADOW
BOXING**

12

Stepping forward on the
right, repeat this double bridge
attack followed by exploding finger
strikes 3 steps forward before #13

劉水功夫遺產在中國

THREE
STEP
ARROW
BOXING

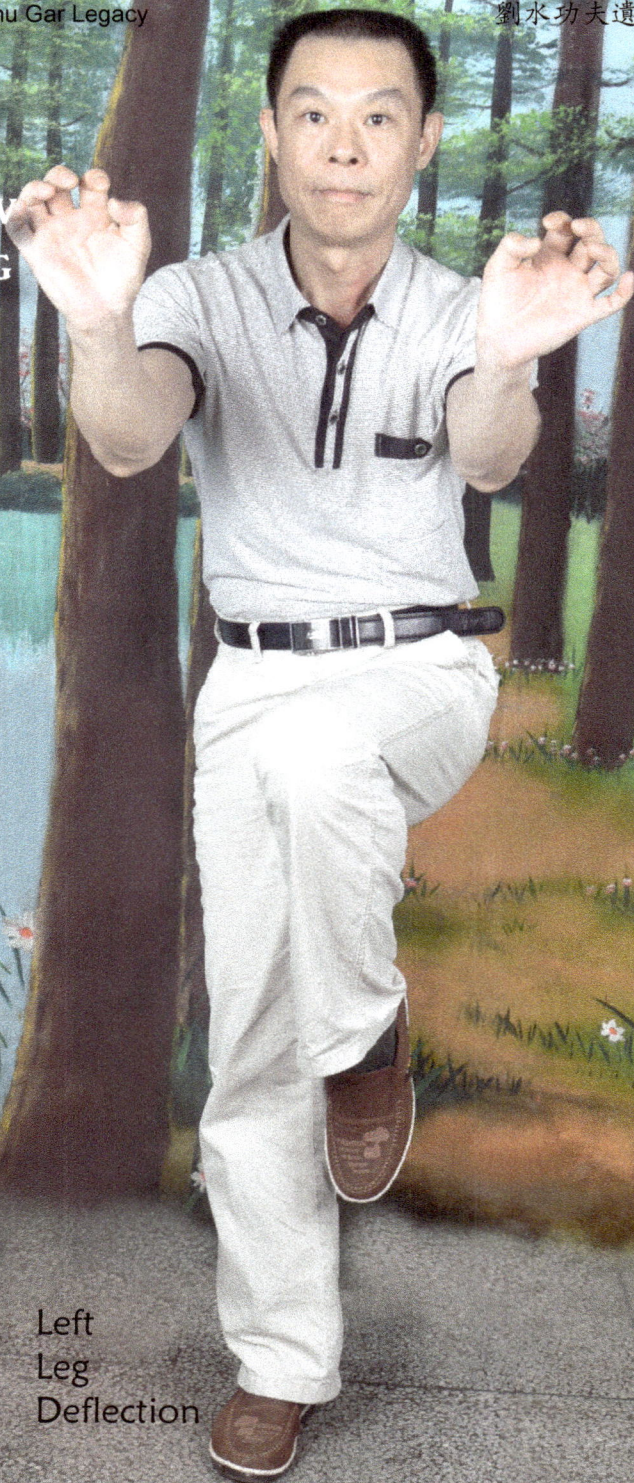

13

Left
Leg
Deflection

三步箭

14

Right
Leg
Deflection

CHU GAR
MANTIS
SHADOW
BOXING

THREE STEP ARROW BOXING

Three Steps forward Phoenix Eye and Finger Strikes, left and right leg deflections are followed by this Gop Sao Clasping Hand

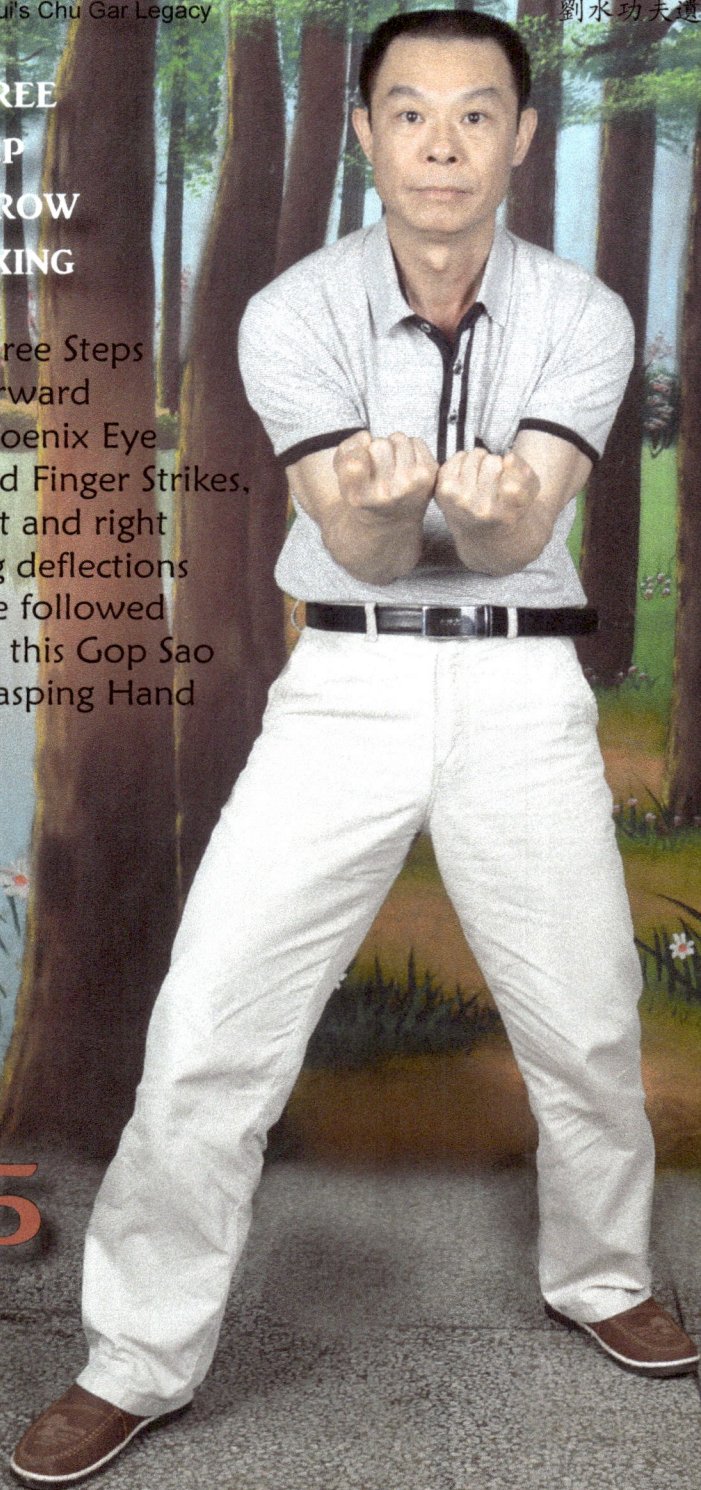

15

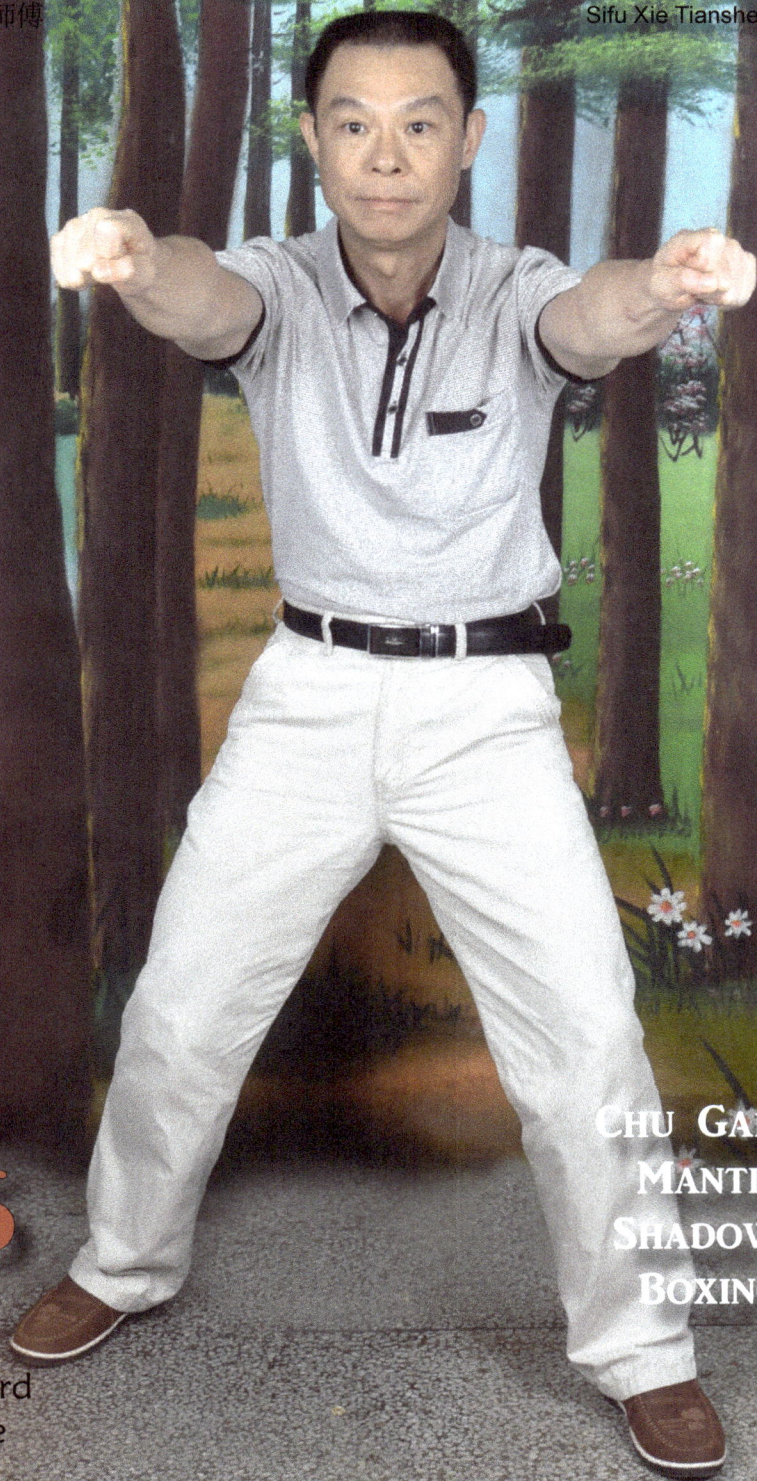

三步箭

16

Step
forward
on the
left

CHU GAR
MANTIS
SHADOW
BOXING

THREE
STEP
ARROW
BOXING

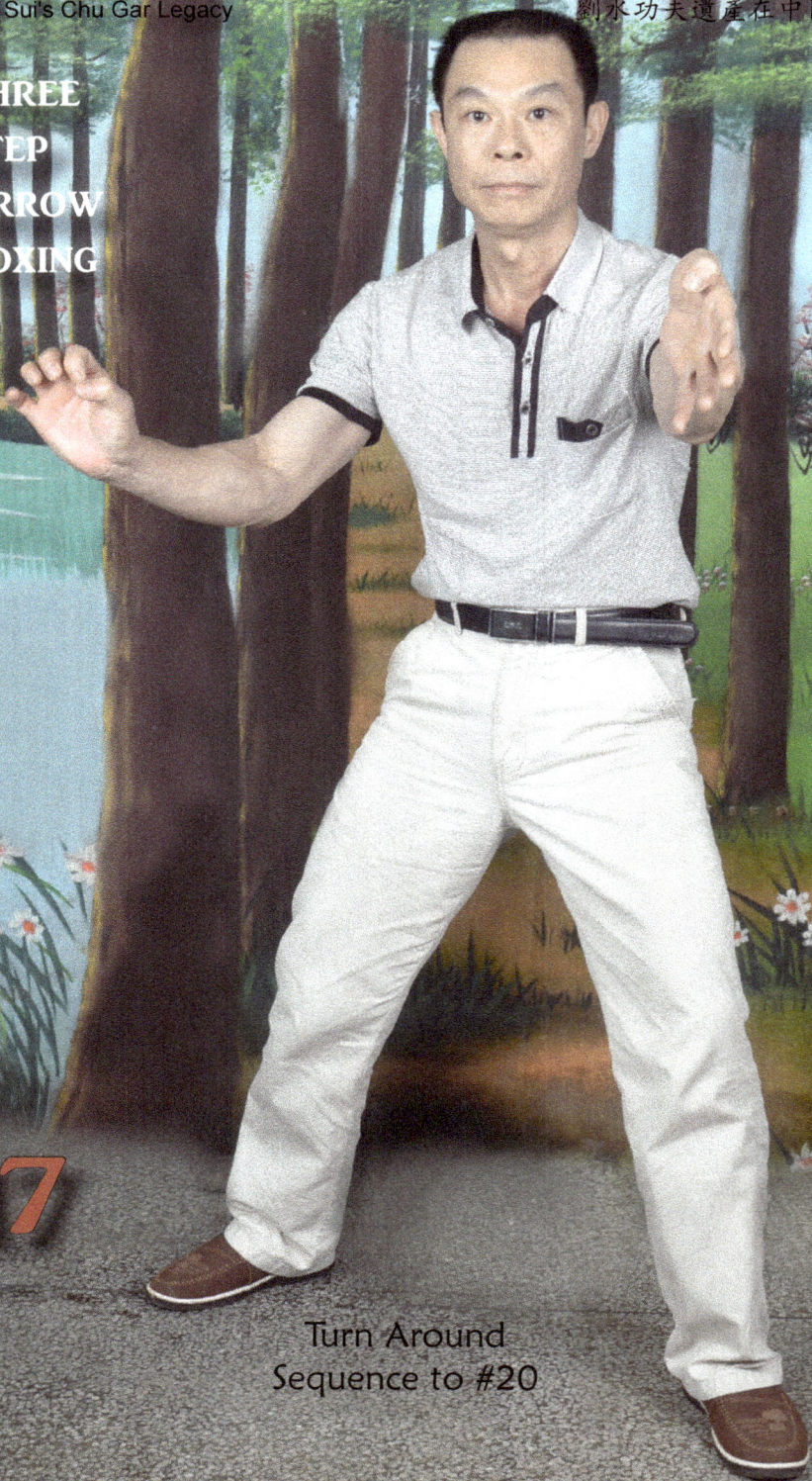

17

Turn Around
Sequence to #20

三步箭

18

CHU GAR
MANTIS
SHADOW
BOXING

Back View

THREE
STEP
ARROW
BOXING

End of
Turn
Around
Sequence

19

Repeat #19 and #20
Three Times as End Sequence

三步箭

20

CHU GAR
MANTIS
SHADOW
BOXING

From #19
Step back and execute #20

劉水功夫遺產在中國

THREE
STEP
ARROW
BOXING

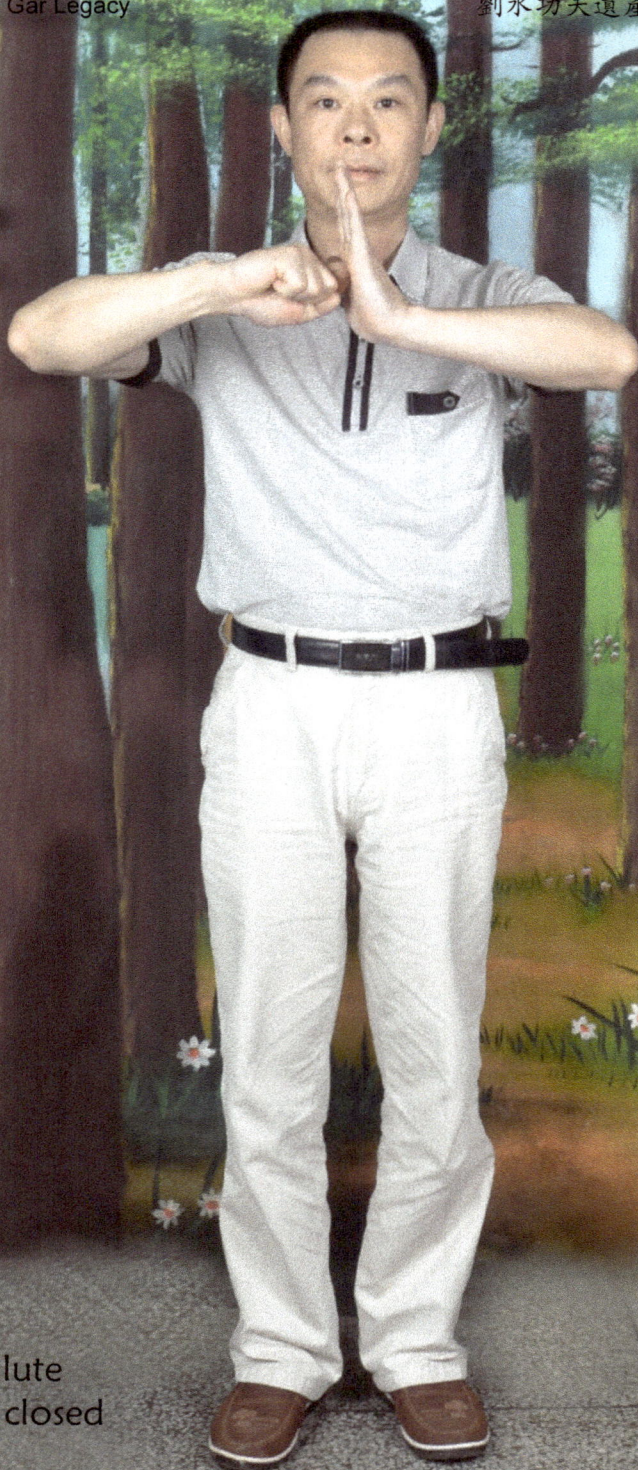

21

Ending salute
with feet closed

THREE
ARROW
三箭搖橋
SHAKING
BRIDGE

Chu Gar Mantis
Shadowboxing Forms

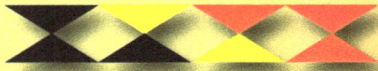

The following pages are a pictorial of the Three Arrow Shaking Bridge boxing form as played in Lao Sui's Village today.

(Refer to the
Southern Mantis Press book, "Chu Gar Gao,"
for more information about the Som Gin Yu Kiu form.)

陳建明師傅

三箭搖橋演示

THREE
ARROWS
SHAKING
BRIDGE
BOXING

Opening
Salute
With
Right
Phoenix
Eye

劉水功夫遺蹤在中國

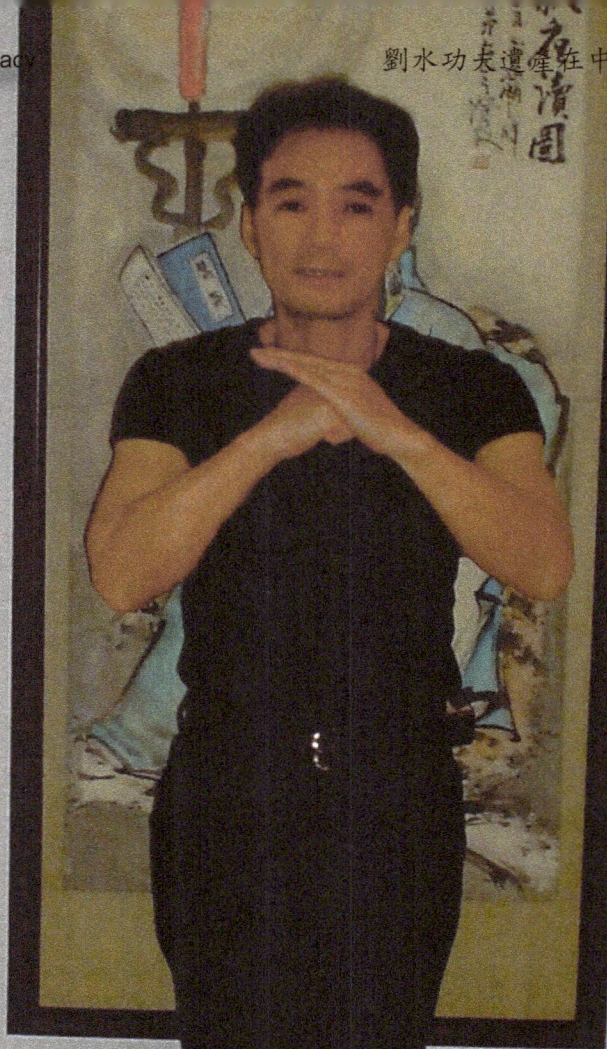

1

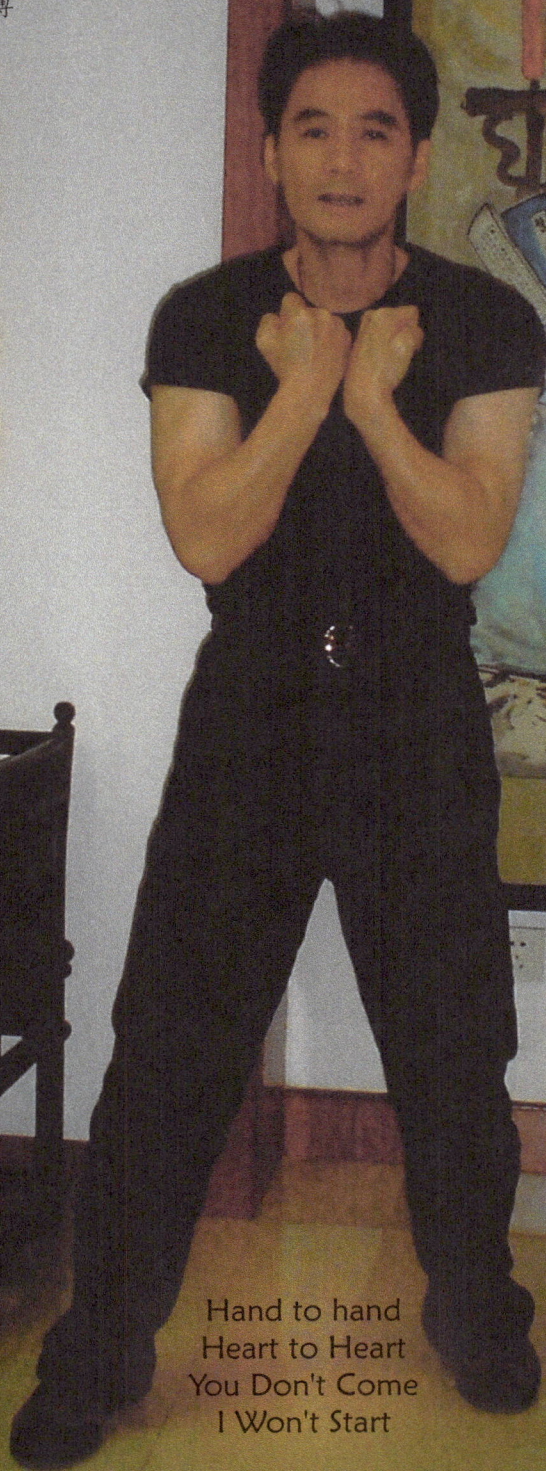

三箭搖橋

陈建明師傅

Sifu Chen Jianming

2

CHU GAR
MANTIS
SHADOW
BOXING

Hand to hand
Heart to Heart
You Don't Come
I Won't Start

劉水功夫遺產在中國

THREE ARROWS SHAKING BRIDGE BOXING

Opening
Sequence
Includes
Postures
#1 - #11

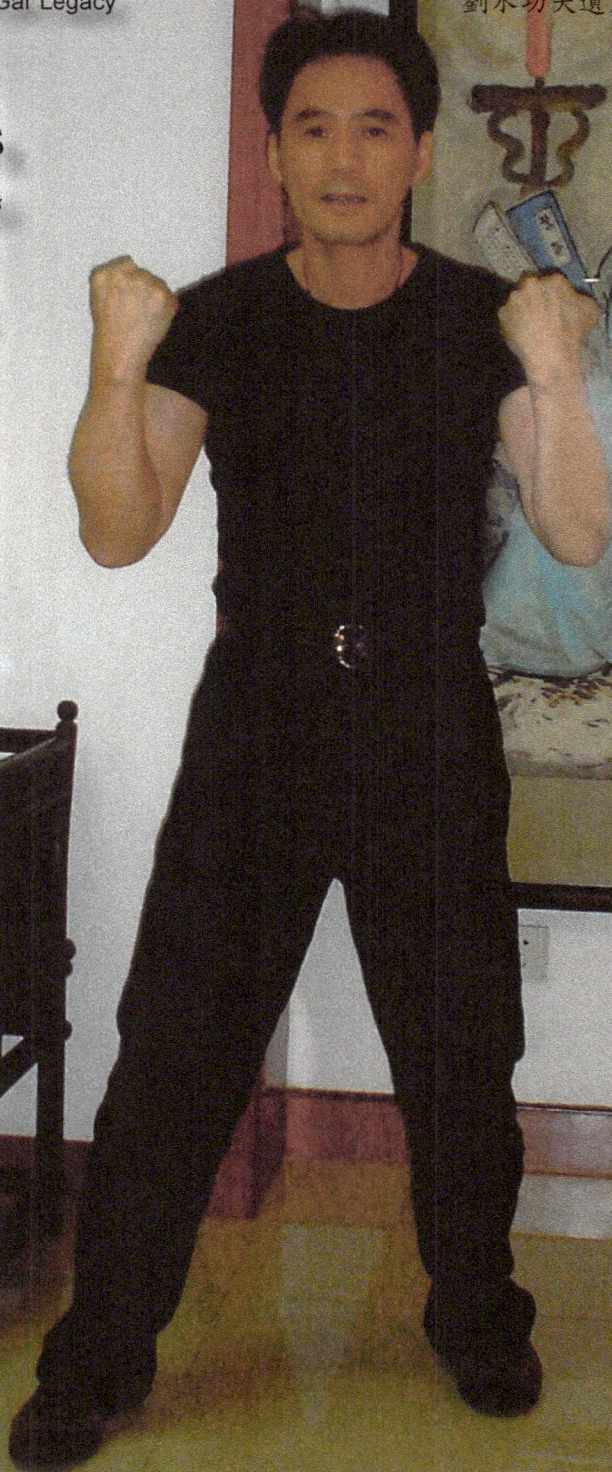

3

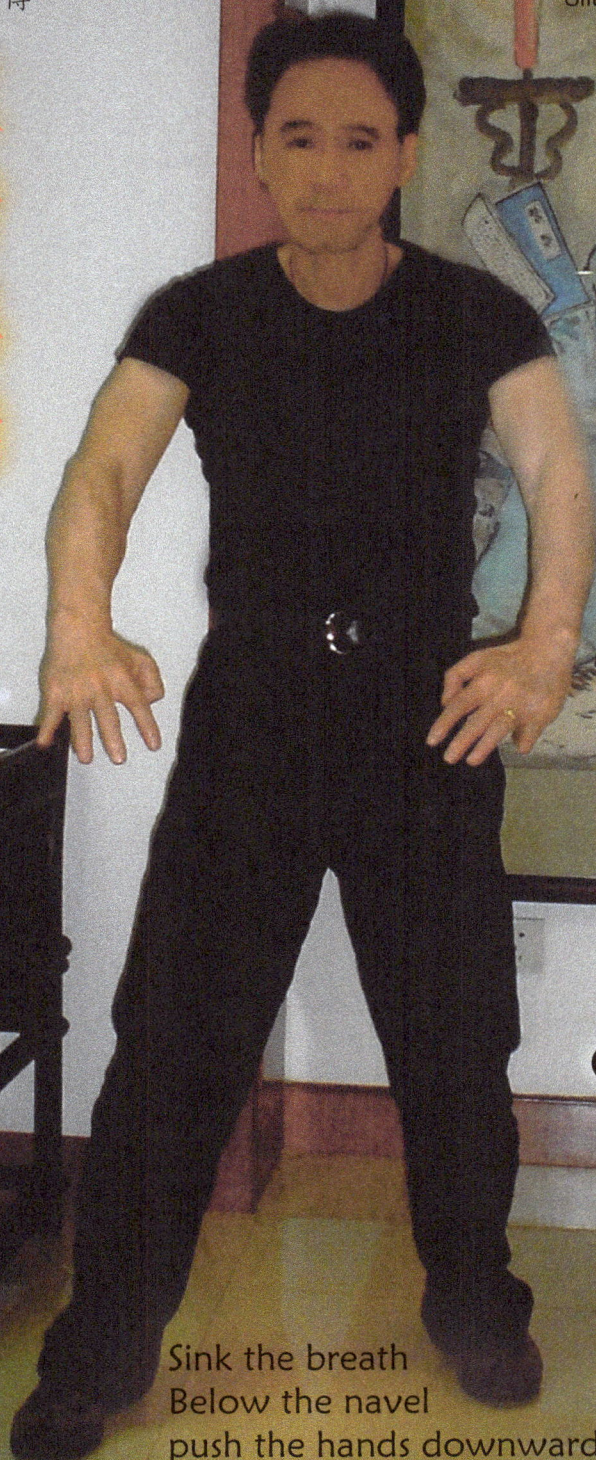

三箭搖橋

4

CHU GAR
MANTIS
SHADOW
BOXING

Sink the breath
Below the navel
push the hands downward

THREE
ARROWS
SHAKING
BRIDGE
BOXING

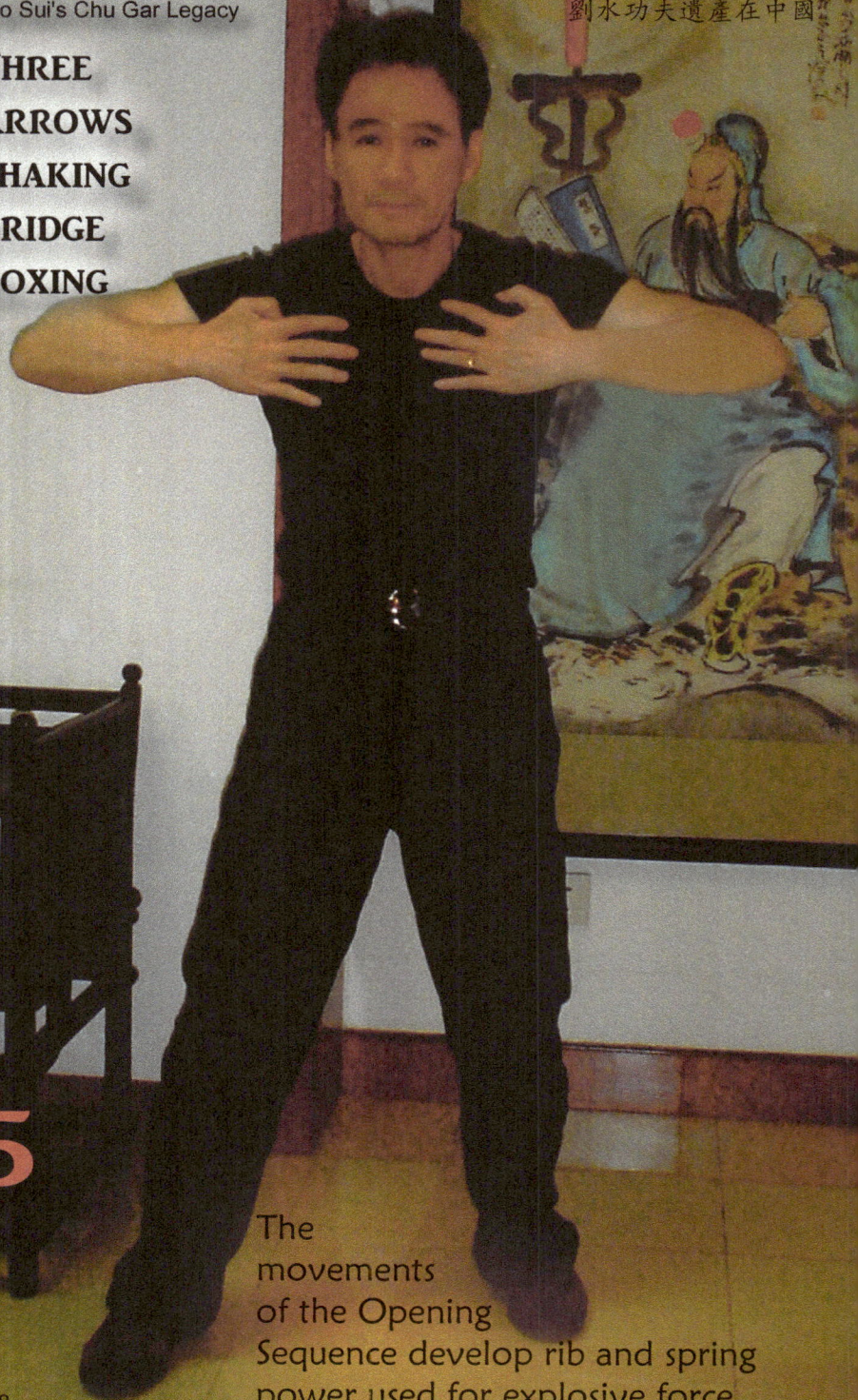

劉水功夫遺產在中國

5

The movements of the Opening Sequence develop rib and spring power used for explosive force

陈建明师傅

三箭搖橋

6

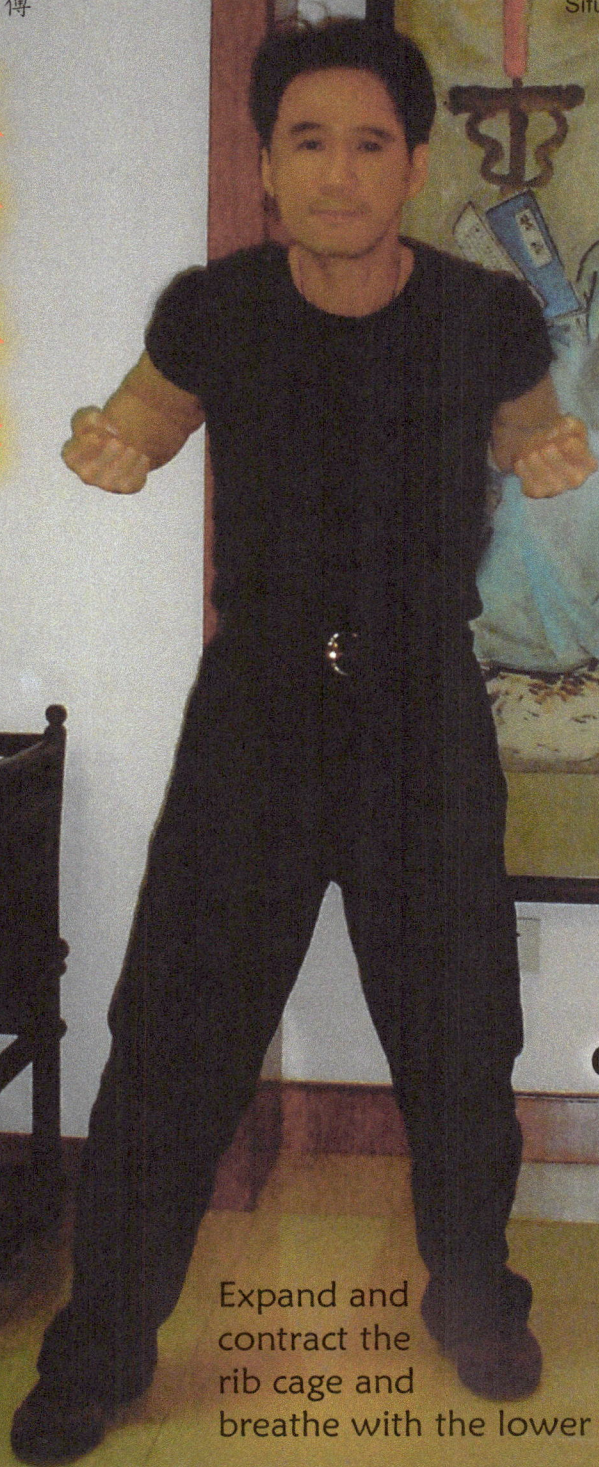

CHU GAR MANTIS SHADOW BOXING

Expand and
contract the
rib cage and
breathe with the lower abdomen

劉水功夫遺產在中國

THREE ARROWS SHAKING BRIDGE BOXING

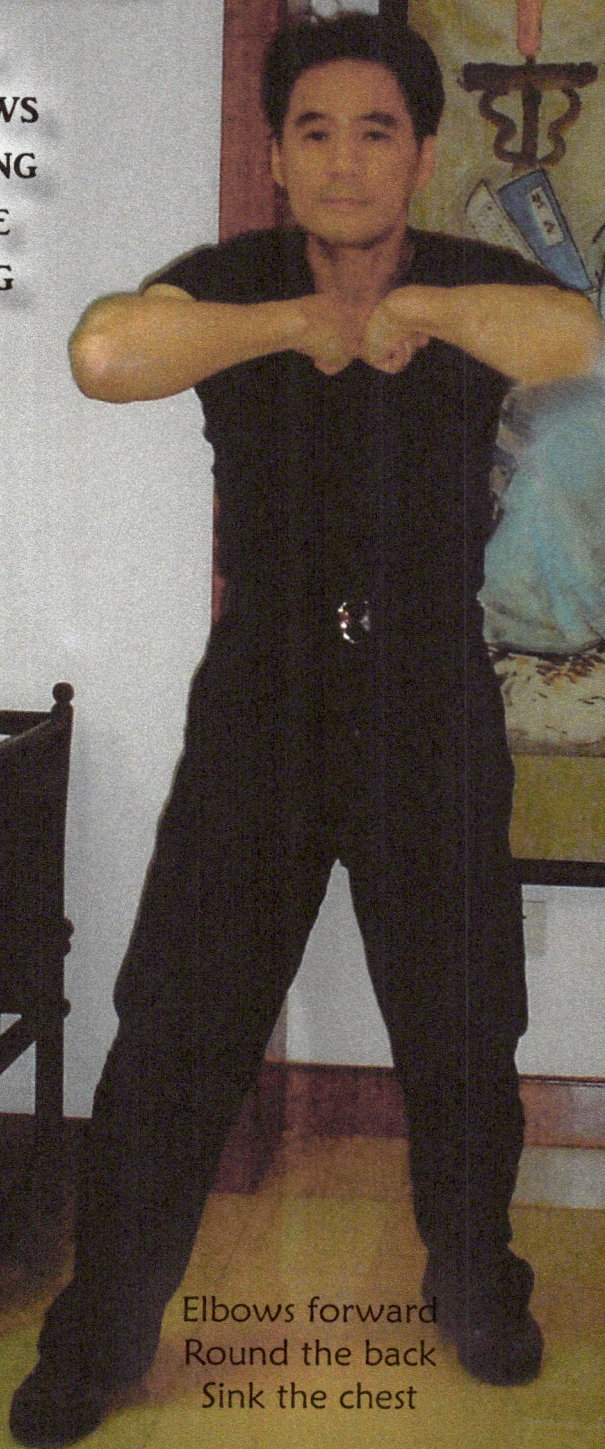

7

Elbows forward
Round the back
Sink the chest

三箭搖橋

8

CHU GAR MANTIS SHADOW BOXING

Inner and
outer
forearms
slice and deflect in all directions

THREE
ARROWS
SHAKING
BRIDGE
BOXING

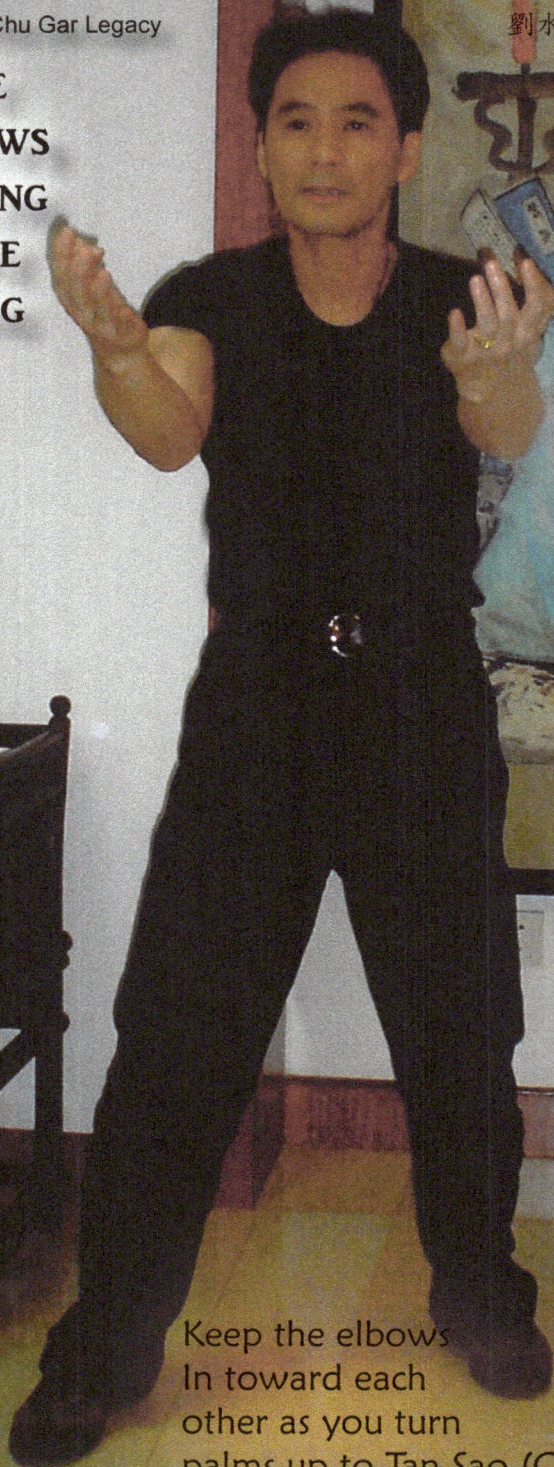

劉水功夫遺產在中國

9

Keep the elbows
In toward each
other as you turn
palms up to Tan Sao (Choc Sao)

Sifu Chen Jianming

三箭搖橋

Quickly turn the palms over and spear the fingers outward stretching from the shoulder

10

CHU GAR
MANTIS
SHADOW
BOXING

Three Arrows Shaking Bridge Boxing

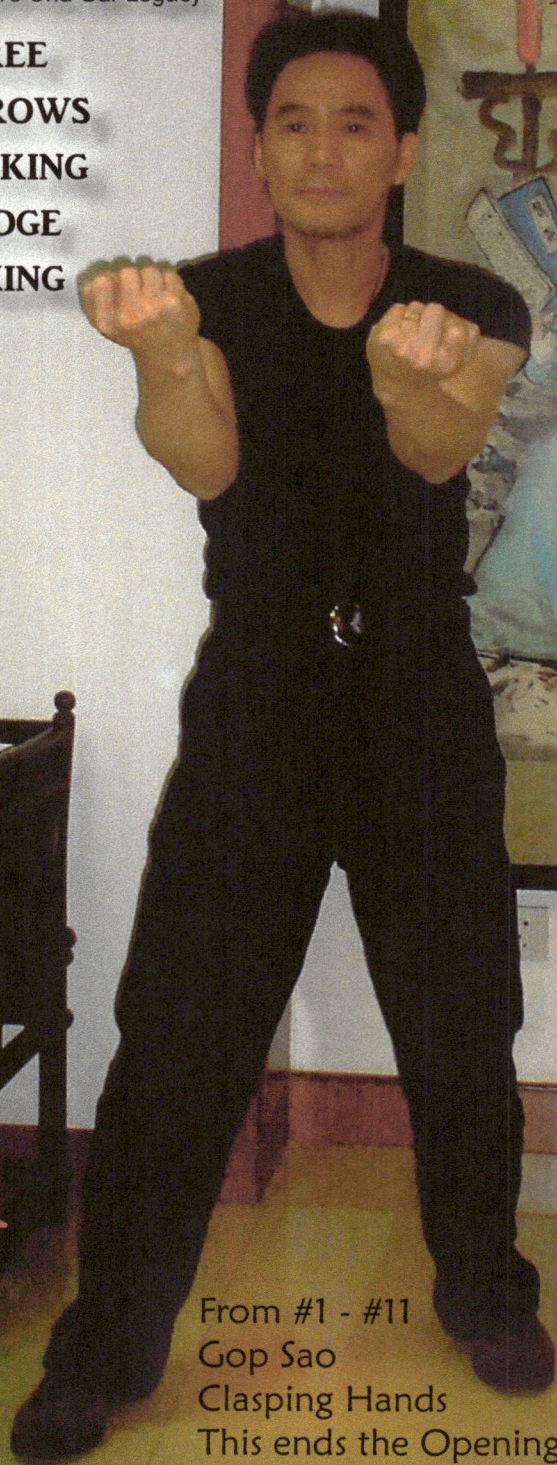

劉水功夫遺產在中國

11

From #1 - #11
Gop Sao
Clasping Hands
This ends the Opening Sequence

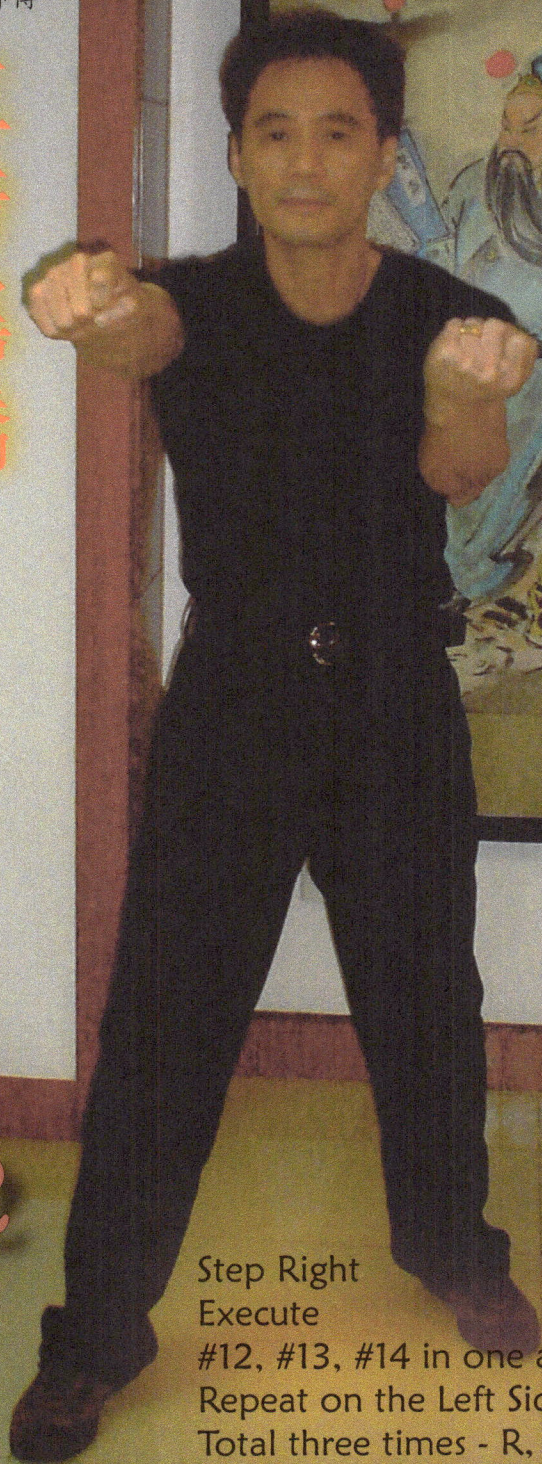

三箭搖橋

**CHU GAR
MANTIS
SHADOW
BOXING**

12

Step Right
Execute
#12, #13, #14 in one action
Repeat on the Left Side & Right Side
Total three times - R, L, R

115

劉水功夫遺產在中國讚同

Spearing
Fingertips

THREE
ARROWS
SHAKING
BRIDGE
BOXING

13

Step Right
Execute
#12, #13, #14
Repeat on the Left Side & Right
Total three times - R, L, R

三箭搖橋

#12, #13, #14
Phoenix Eye Punch
Fingertip Spear
Gop Sao
In
3 Steps
R, L, R

One Step
Three Actions
#12, #13, #14

CHU GAR
MANTIS
SHADOW
BOXING

14

Step Right
Execute
#12, #13, #14
Repeat on the Left Side & Right
Total three times - R, L, R

劉水功夫遺產在中國

THREE
ARROWS
SHAKING
BRIDGE
BOXING

15

Left
Leg
Deflection

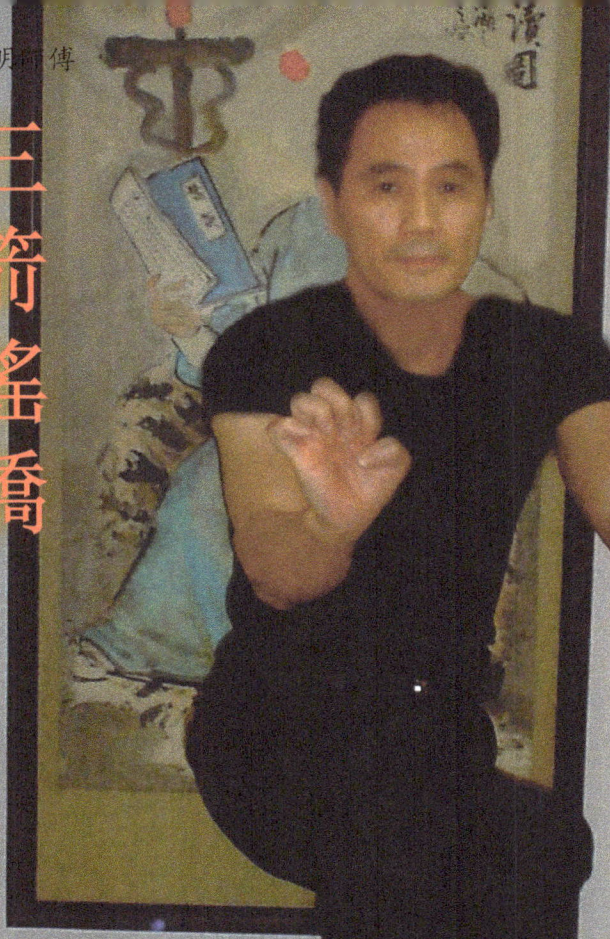

三箭搖橋

CHU GAR
MANTIS
SHADOW
BOXING

16

Right
Leg
Deflection

劉水功夫遺產在中國

THREE
ARROWS
SHAKING
BRIDGE
BOXING

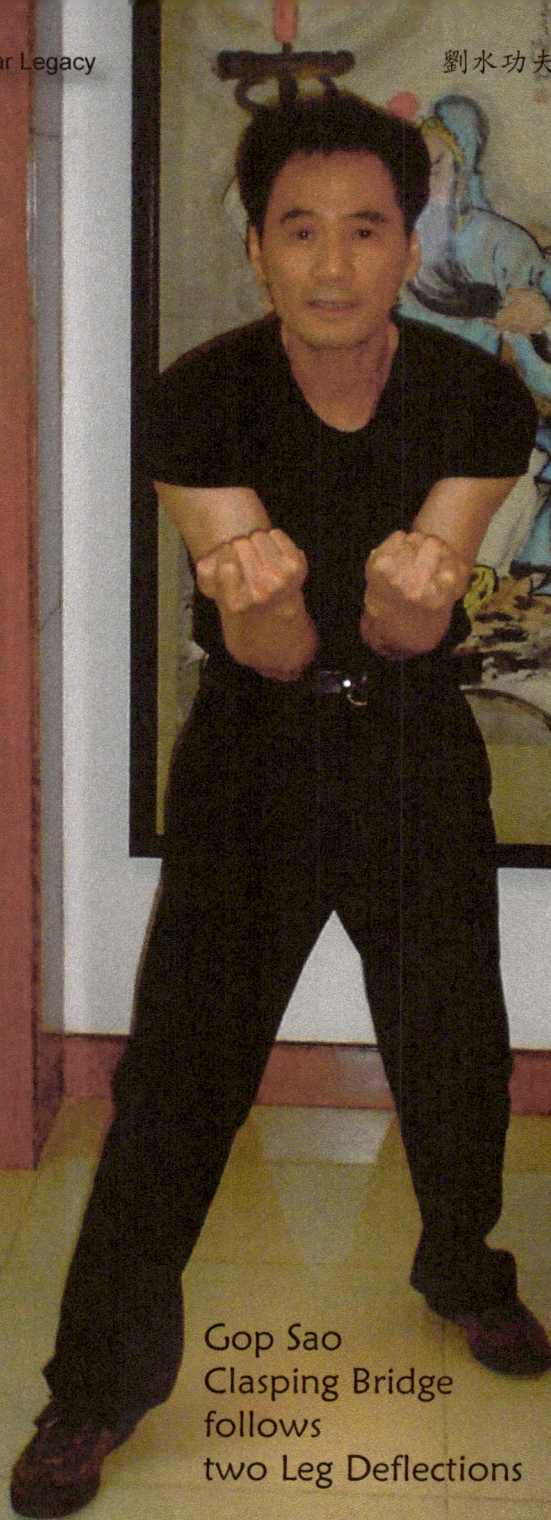

17

Gop Sao
Clasping Bridge
follows
two Leg Deflections

三箭搖橋

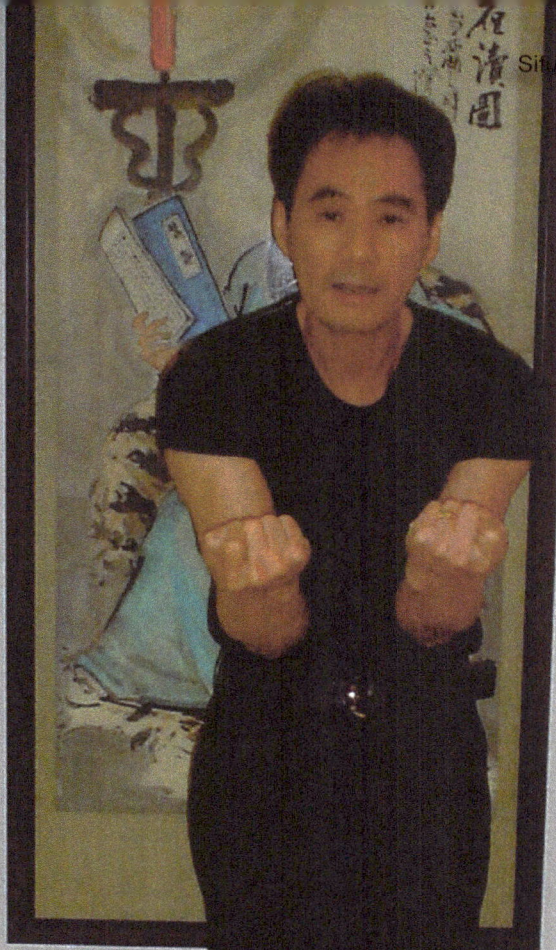

CHU GAR
MANTIS
SHADOW
BOXING

18

Right leg
back to left leg
begin turn around
sequence

THREE ARROWS SHAKING BRIDGE BOXING

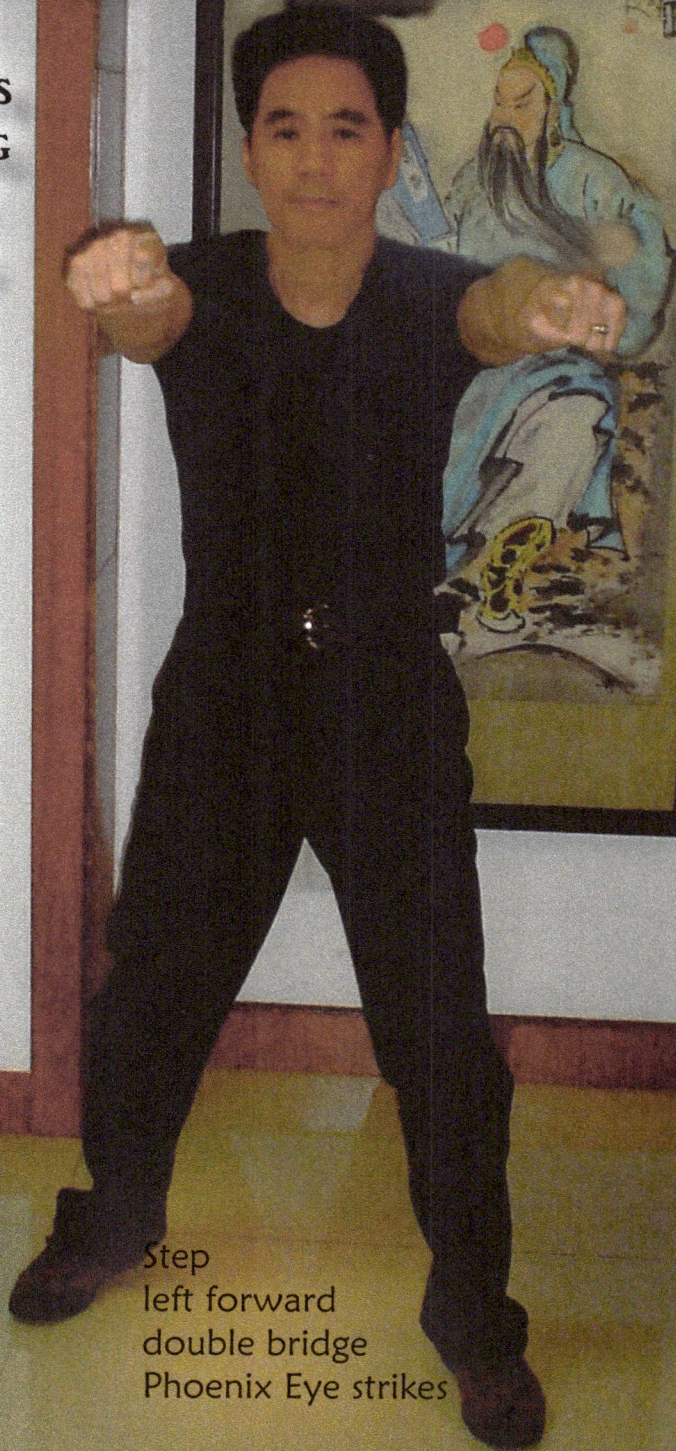

劉水功夫遺產在中國

19

Step
left forward
double bridge
Phoenix Eye strikes

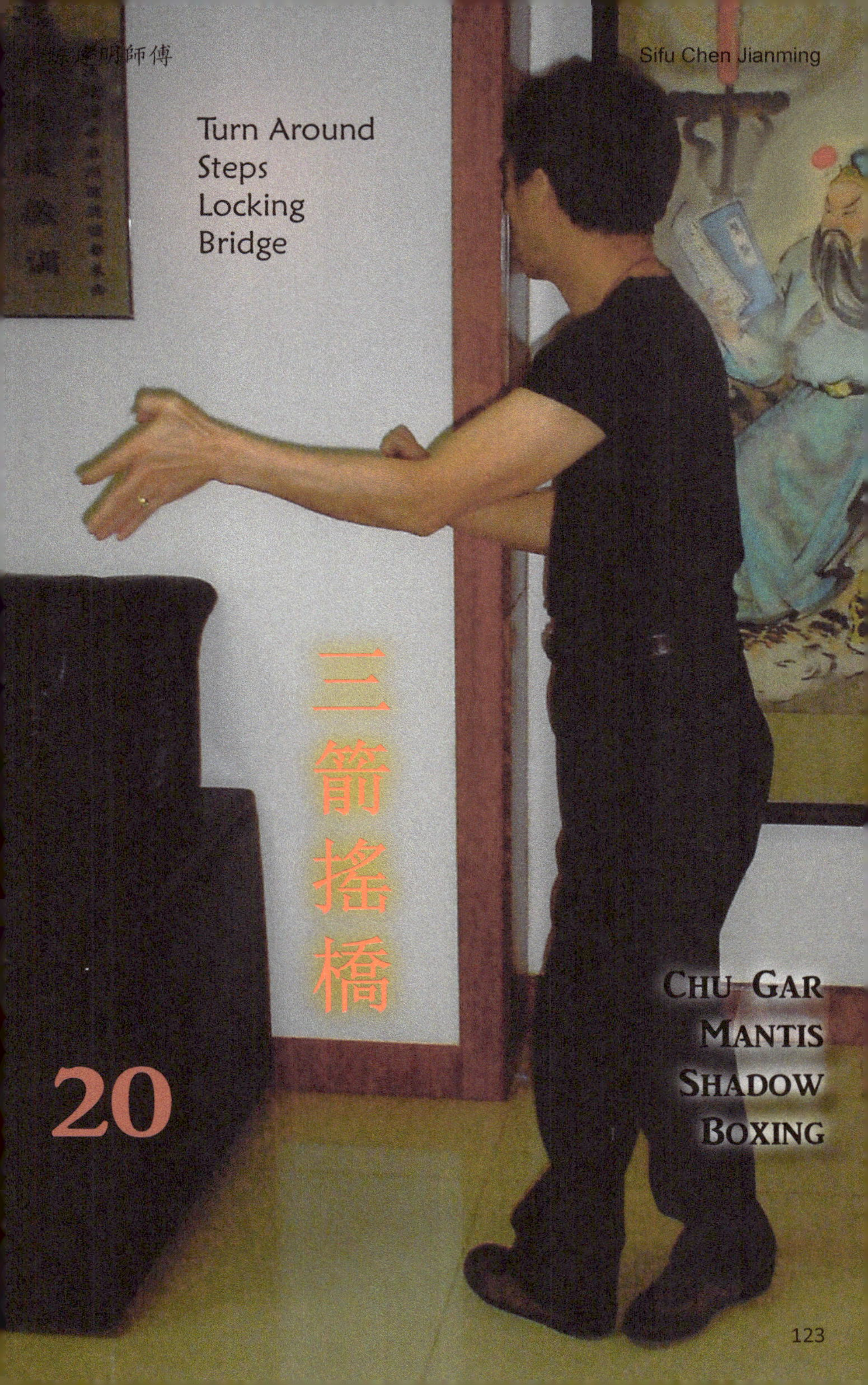

Turn Around
Steps
Locking
Bridge

三箭搖橋

20

CHU GAR
MANTIS
SHADOW
BOXING

劉水功夫遺產在中國

THREE ARROWS SHAKING BRIDGE BOXING

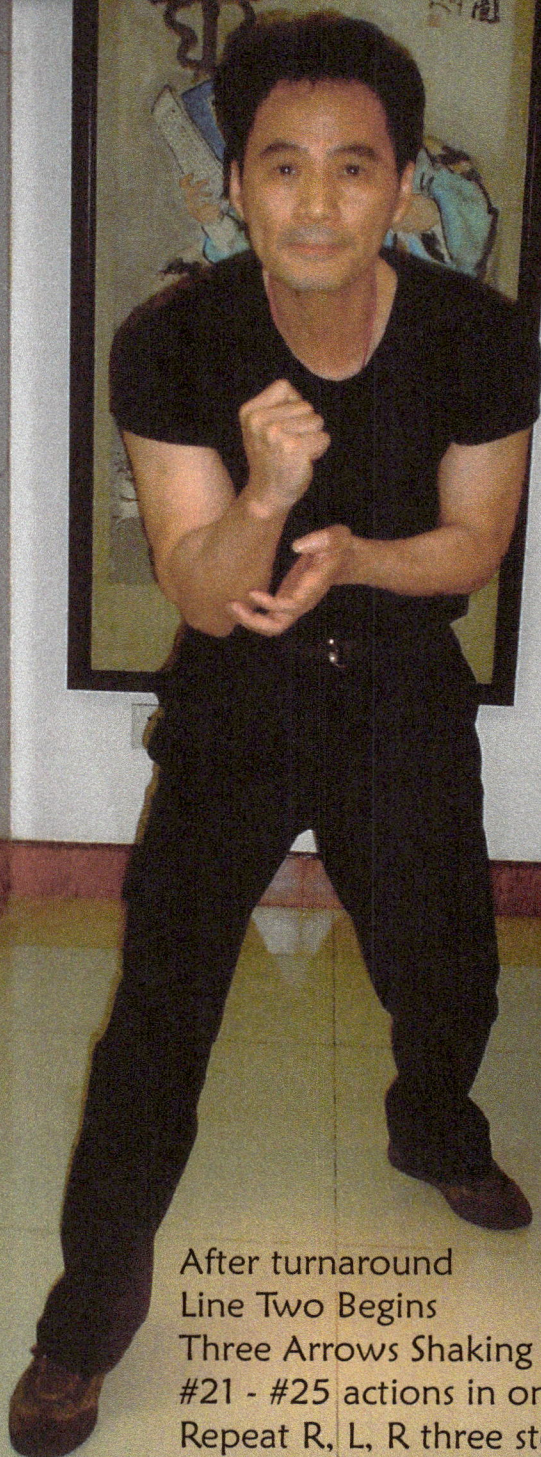

21

After turnaround
Line Two Begins
Three Arrows Shaking Bridge
#21 - #25 actions in one step
Repeat R, L, R three steps

三箭搖橋

CHU GAR MANTIS SHADOW BOXING

22

Three Arrows Shaking Bridge
#21 - #25 actions in one step
Repeat R, L, R three steps

THREE ARROWS SHAKING BRIDGE BOXING

劉永功夫遺產在中國

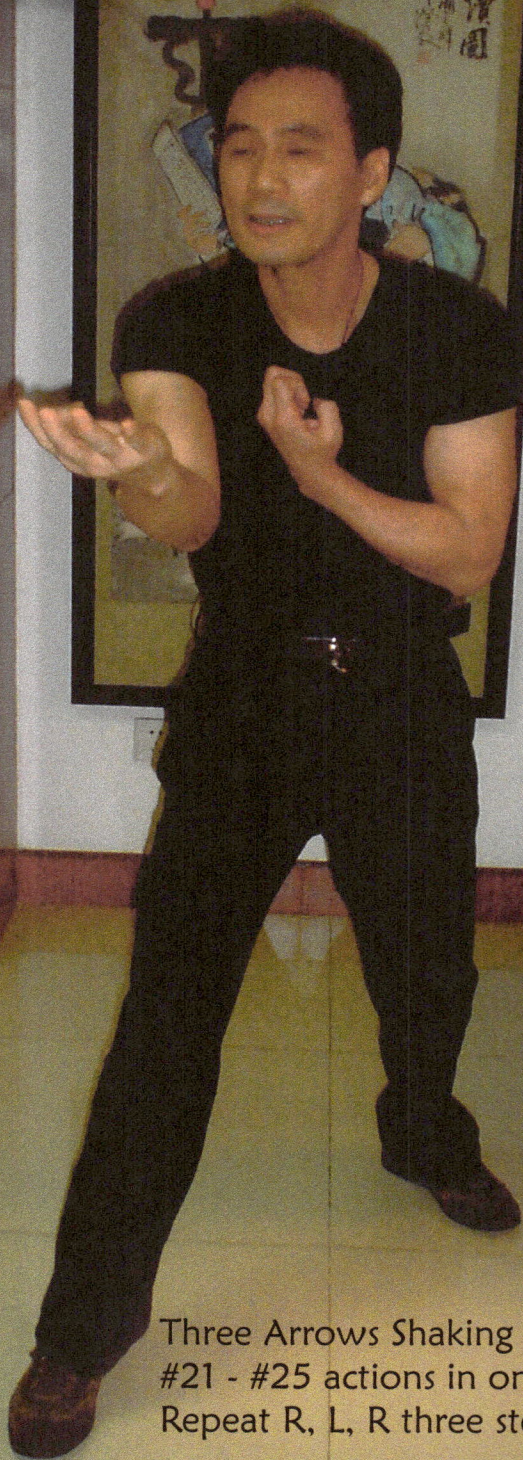

23

Three Arrows Shaking Bridge
#21 - #25 actions in one step
Repeat R, L, R three steps

126

三箭搖橋

CHU GAR
MANTIS
SHADOW
BOXING

24

Three Arrows Shaking Bridge
#21 - #25 actions in one step
Repeat R, L, R three steps

THREE ARROWS SHAKING BRIDGE BOXING

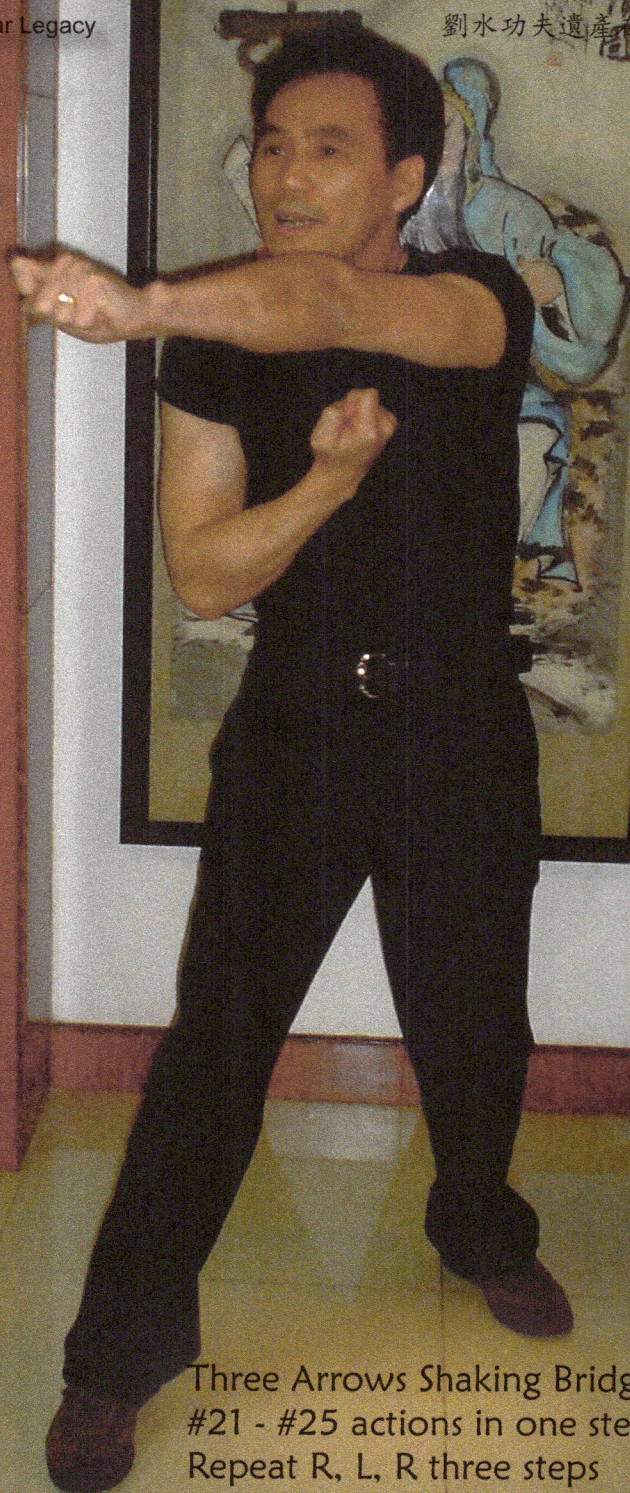

劉水功夫遺產在中國

25

Three Arrows Shaking Bridge
#21 - #25 actions in one step
Repeat R, L, R three steps

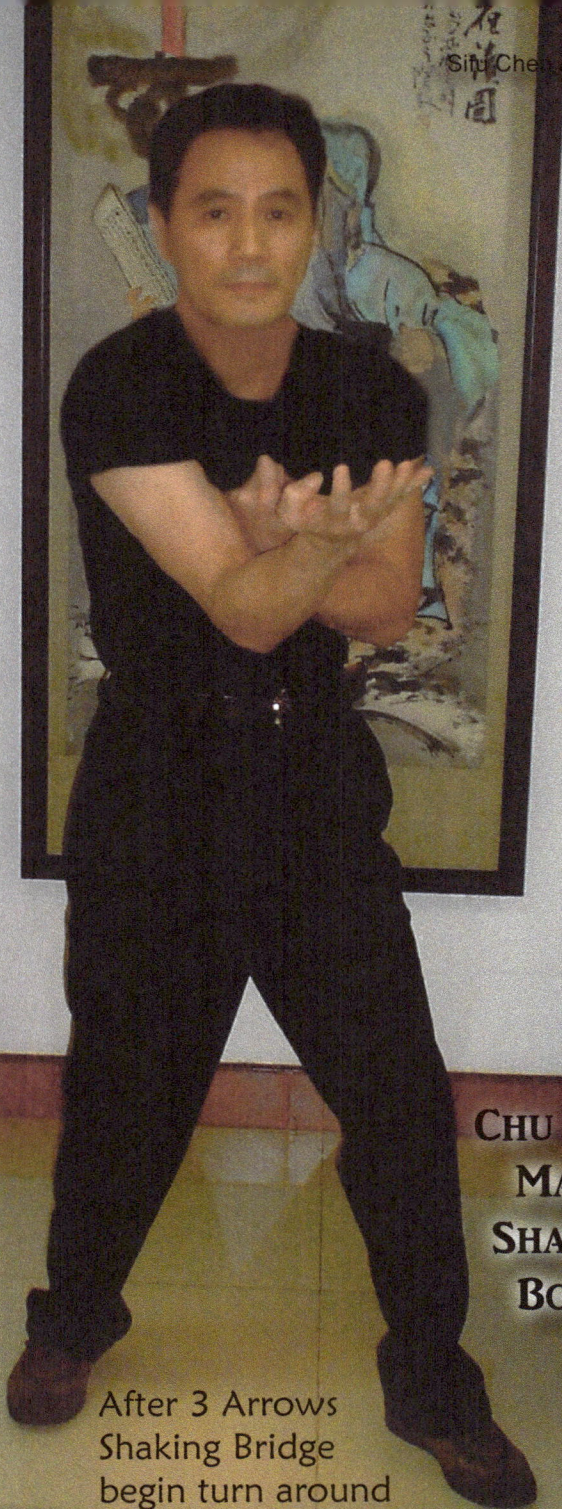

三箭搖橋

26

CHU GAR
MANTIS
SHADOW
BOXING

After 3 Arrows
Shaking Bridge
begin turn around

劉水功夫遺產在中國

THREE
ARROWS
SHAKING
BRIDGE
BOXING

27

Turn
Around
Steps

三箭搖橋

Double Bridge Fingertip Spearing

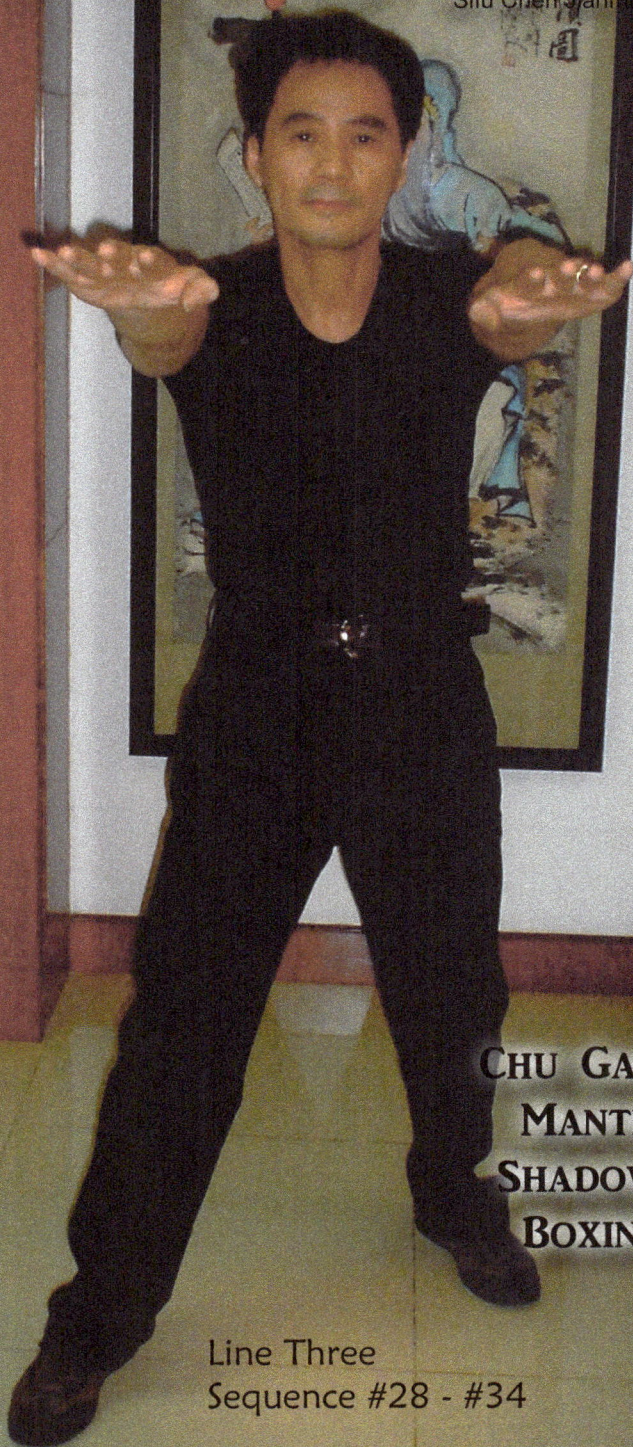

28

CHU GAR
MANTIS
SHADOW
BOXING

Line Three
Sequence #28 - #34

THREE ARROWS SHAKING BRIDGE BOXING

劉水功夫遺產在中國

Bao
Zhuang
close
the
doors

29

Line Three
Sequence #28 - #34

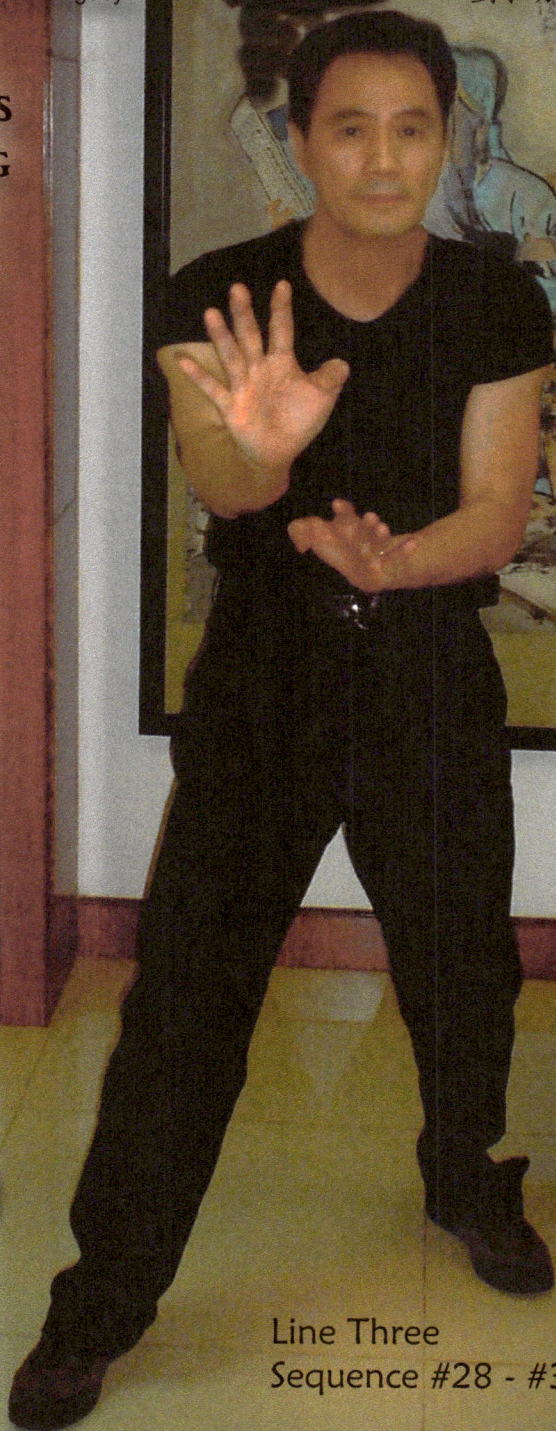

132

三箭搖橋

Fic
Sao
ward
Off

30

CHU GAR
MANTIS
SHADOW
BOXING

Line Three
Sequence #28 - #34

133

劉水功夫遺產在中國

THREE ARROWS SHAKING BRIDGE BOXING

Bao
Zhuang
close
the
doors

31

Line Three
Sequence #28 - #34

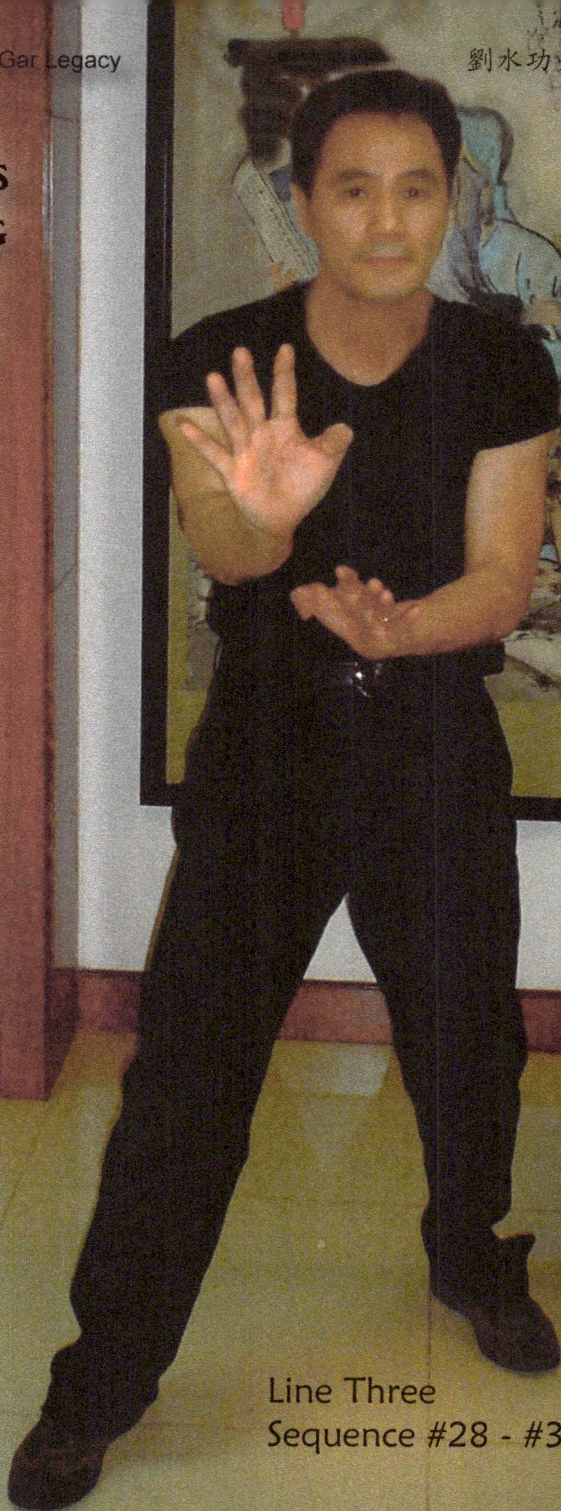

三箭搖橋

Double Bridge Tan Sao

32

CHU GAR
MANTIS
SHADOW
BOXING

Line Three
Sequence #28 - #34

135

THREE ARROWS SHAKING BRIDGE BOXING

Double
Bridge
Fingertip
Spearing

劉水功夫遺產在中國

33

Line Three
Sequence #28 - #34

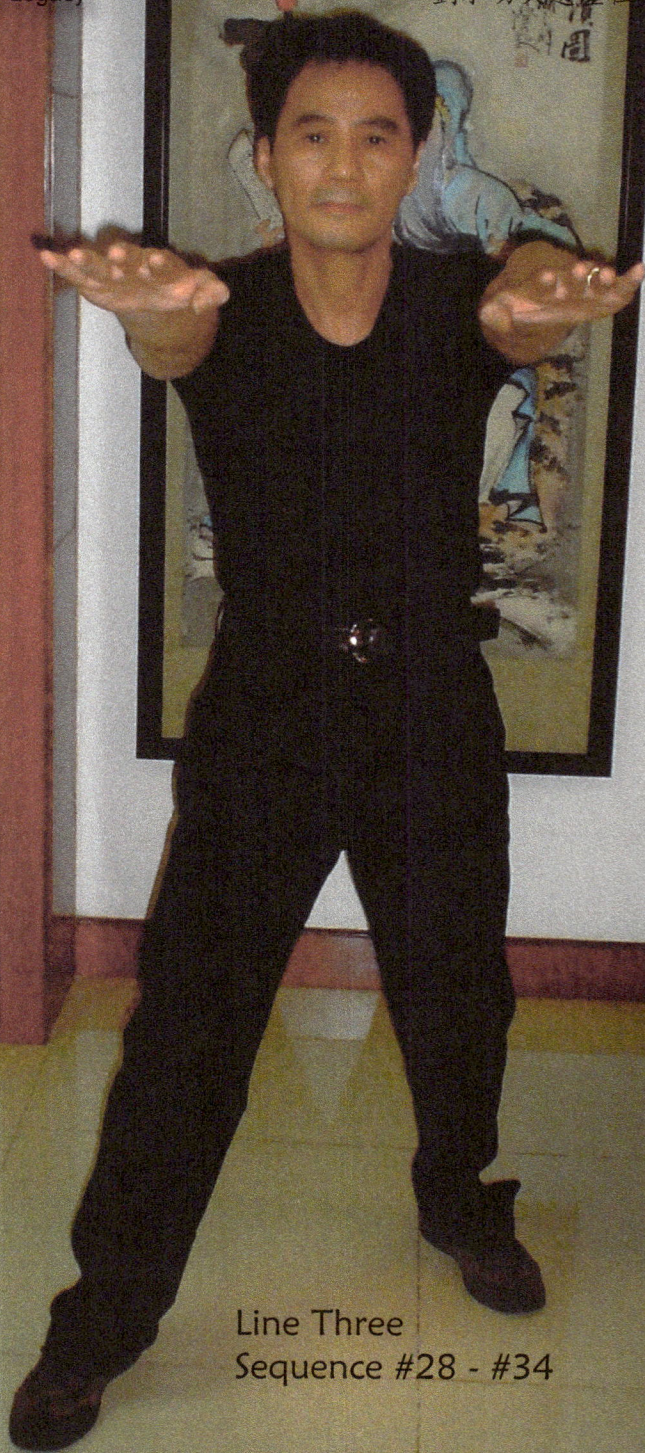

三箭搖橋

Lop Sao
Double
Grasping
Step Back

34

CHU GAR
MANTIS
SHADOW
BOXING

Line Three
Sequence #28 - #34

THREE ARROWS SHAKING BRIDGE BOXING

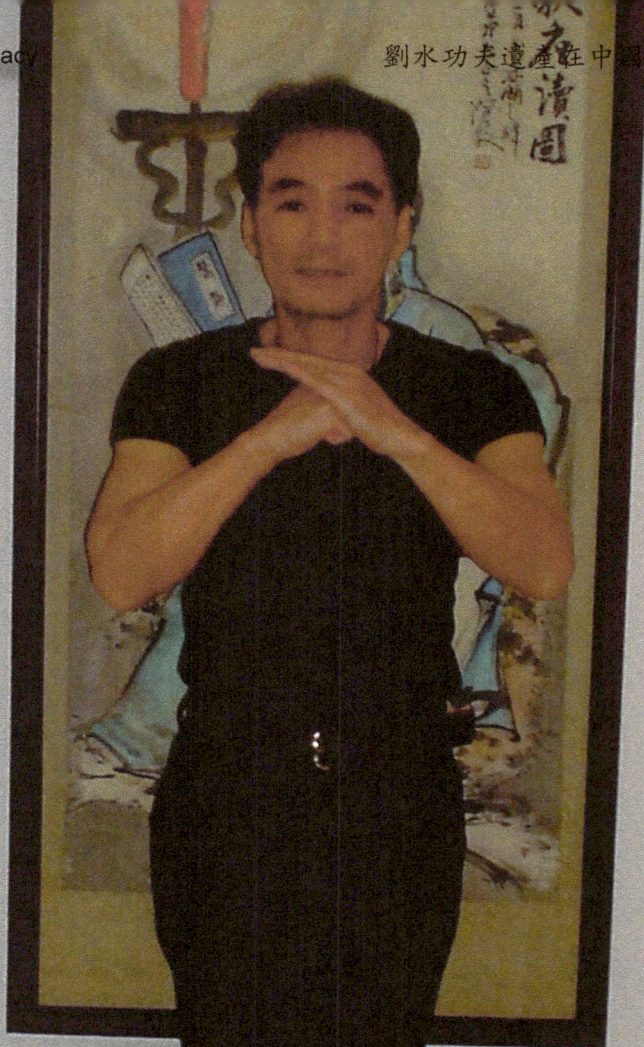

劉水功夫遺產在中國

35

End Salute

**Images from
Lao Sui's Hometown**

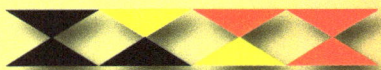

劉水的故鄉香園村

劉水功夫遺產在中國

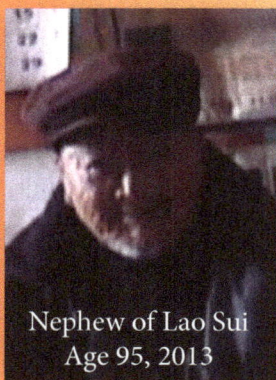

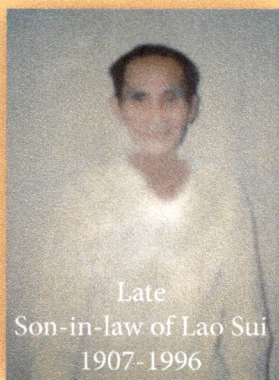

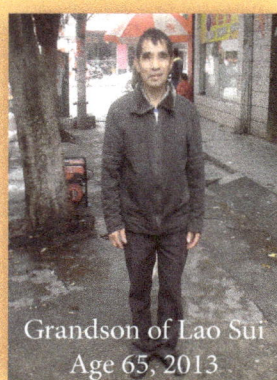

Nephew of Lao Sui
Age 95, 2013

Late
Son-in-law of Lao Sui
1907-1996

Grandson of Lao Sui
Age 65, 2013

L–R) LAO XIANG NAN, MA MING SEN, MA SAO NAN

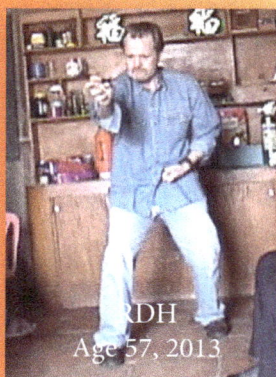

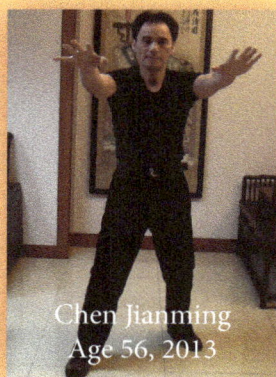

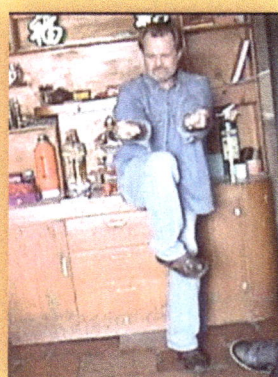

RDH
Age 57, 2013

Chen Jianming
Age 56, 2013

LAO SUI'S CHU GAR MANTIS LEGACY IN CHINA

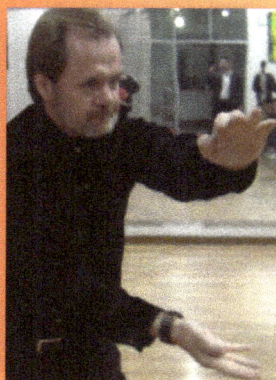

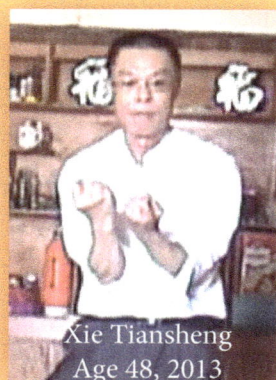

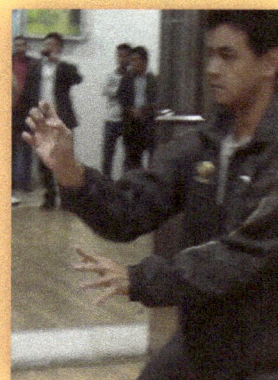

Xie Tiansheng
Age 48, 2013

SIFU CHEN JIANMING'S CHU GAR MANTIS IN HUICHENG

CHINA SOUTHERN MANTIS SURVEY™

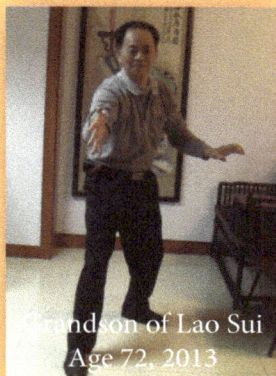

Grandson of Lao Sui
Age 72, 2013

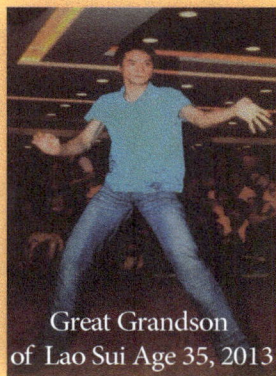

Great Grandson
of Lao Sui Age 35, 2013

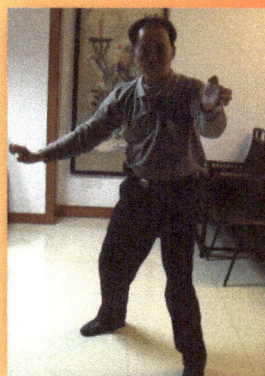

SIFU MA JIUHUA AND THE LAO FAMILY KIN

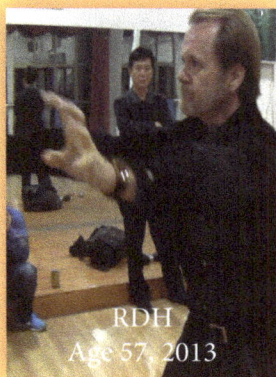

RDH
Age 57, 2013

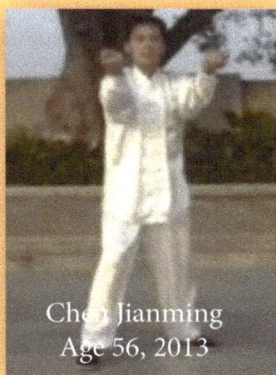

Chen Jianming
Age 56, 2013

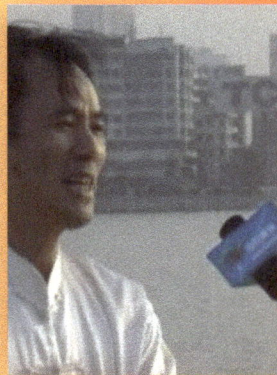

中國南螳螂功夫專題訪查

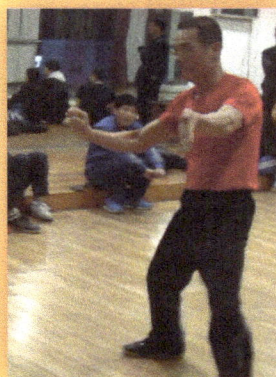

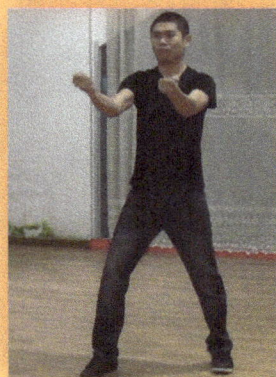

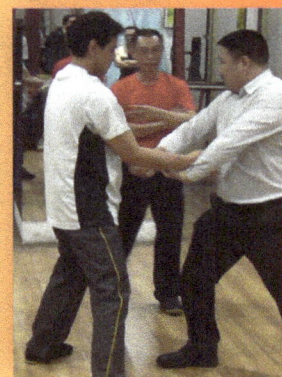

SIFU XIE TIANSHENG'S CHU GAR MANTIS IN BOLUO

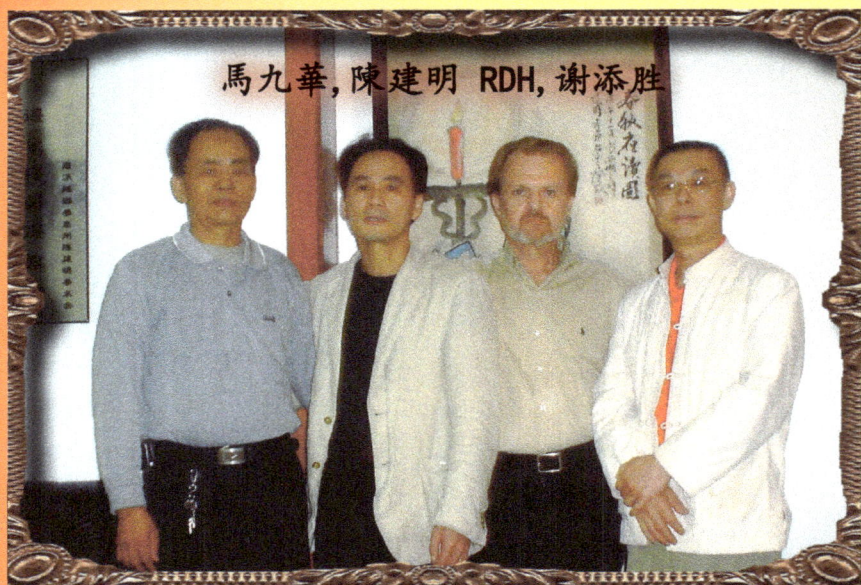

馬九華, 陳建明 RDH, 謝添胜

Above: Ma Jiuhua, Chen Jianming, RDH, Xie Tiansheng
Below: RDH exchanges with Xie Tiansheng Clan
下圖: RDH, 與 謝添勝, 及其弟子武術交流

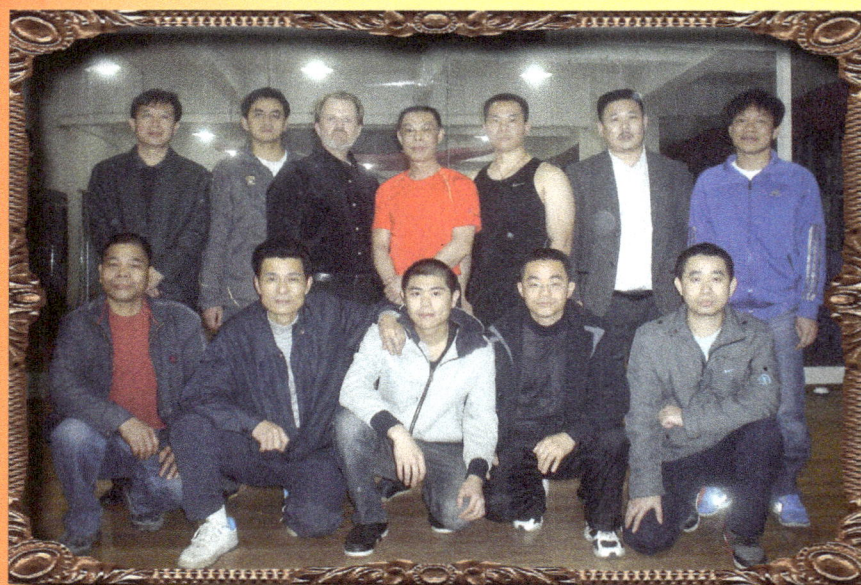

由左至右：謝添勝、馬九華、RDH、劉健強、張庭

Left to Right)
Xie Tiansheng, Ma Jiuhua, RDH, Lao Jian Chang, Zhang Ting

1936 年在香港的劉水匯款在他的家鄉惠陽縣營建新屋，但他從未能親眼目睹新屋落成，時至今日，它依然是他的後人、朋友和鄰居的故居。

In 1936, while living in Hong Kong, Lao Sui financed in his hometown, Huiyang, Huizhou, this house. He was never able to return home and never saw the house. Today, it is still home to his family, friends, and neighbors.

143

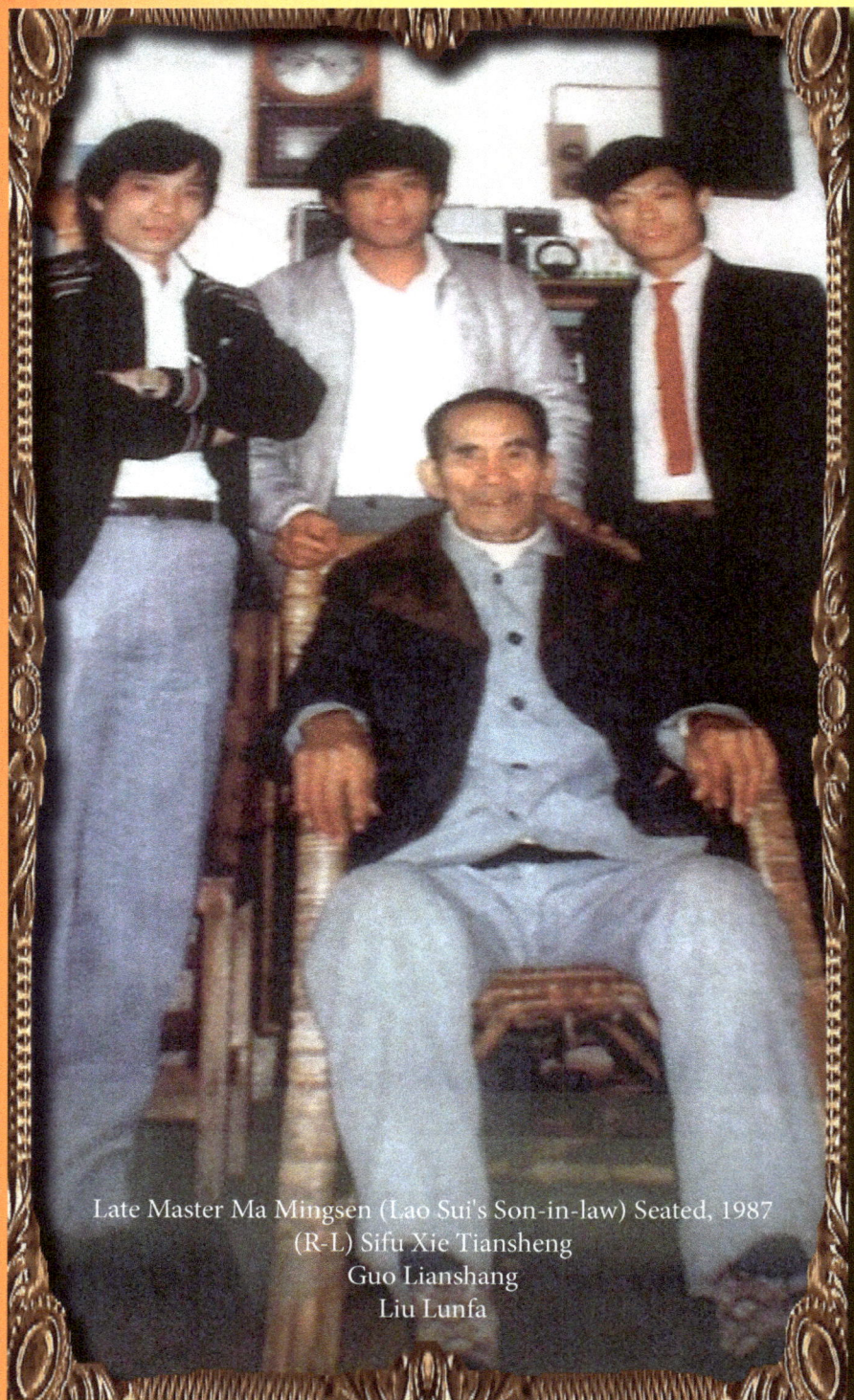

Late Master Ma Mingsen (Lao Sui's Son-in-law) Seated, 1987
(R-L) Sifu Xie Tiansheng
Guo Lianshang
Liu Lunfa

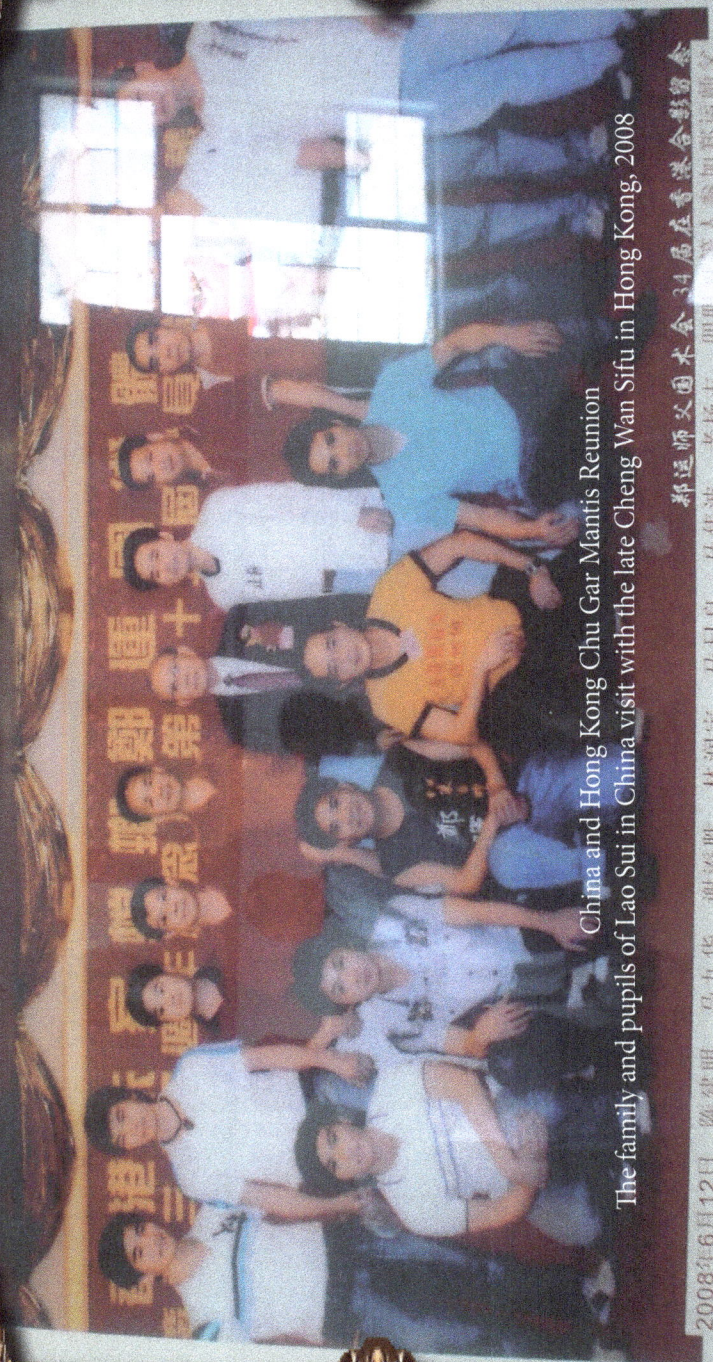

China and Hong Kong Chu Gar Mantis Reunion

The family and pupils of Lao Sui in China visit with the late Cheng Wan Sifu in Hong Kong, 2008

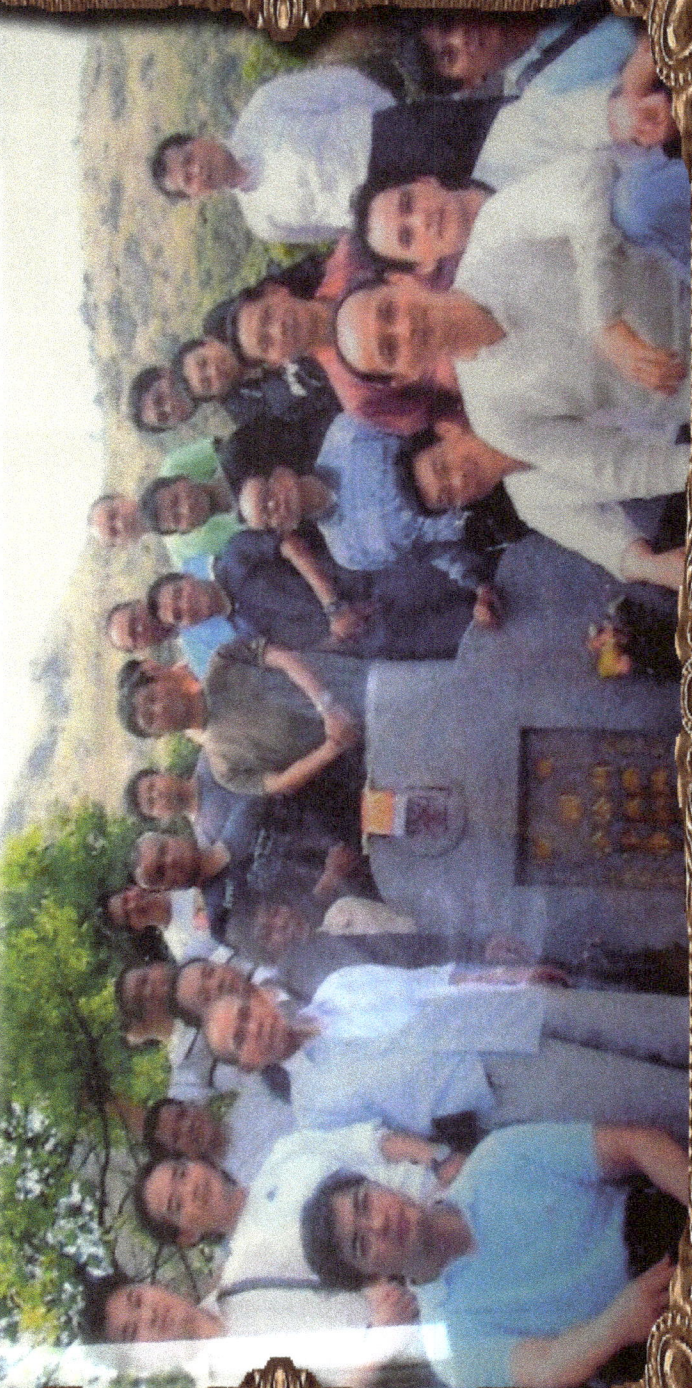

2009年清明节香港剑师公墓合照

The family and pupils of Lao Sui in China and Hong Kong visit Lao Sui's Hong Kong tomb, 2009

劉水軼事
Lao Sui Lore

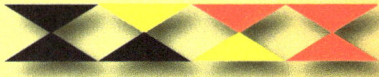

A small exhibition gallery in Lao Sui's village today
displays his existing writings as well as photographs
and written history about Chu Gar Southern Praying Mantis.
The following pages detail a few (refer to page 62).

一個展示館位於劉水的故鄉香園村
展示他的手稿以及照片

和關於朱家螳螂歷史的文獻。

在下文中列舉數項 （請參閱第 62 頁）

南派东江螳螂拳简介

　　南派螳螂拳始创于清中叶，至今已有两百多年历史，始创人为南少林俗事朱（周）亚南祖师，广东嘉应州（今兴宁人氏世业农，为土富。年少时因患胃病，四处求医无效，其父之友疑与水土有关，劝其远行易环境，希遇名医，否则无望，亚南其父认为有理，便给予亚南资金，使仆人周容相随，令习商贾，不论何处，皆可随意而为。于是亚南拜别家人，沿粤北上，历经湘鄂入赣闽因生活无则，其随仆周容，以年老故，不堪风尘仆仆，亦不支卧病，经月余诊治，不但未愈，继而一命归西，亚南料理丧事后，已床头金尽，急挥书信家中告急，但远水不能救近火，居于目前生活状况，亚南倍感惶恐，幸亏客舍主人，袁翁（大善之人）知其经济之危借于则金，介绍亚南前往南少林寺知客僧禅隐大师处，诊治胃病，此僧乃得道之人，精医术，得少林真传，武高深不可测，与客舍主人袁翁关系甚好，经禅隐大师的诊治亚南的病不久便获痊愈，但因离家较远，亚南也为其现状，生活担忧，店主袁翁洞悉其意，便问亚南愿否在少林寺谋份差事，其日后生活也可看落，亚南便答不论任何苦差也愿任之，袁店主便告挚友禅隐大师亦表示同情。允许其以炊事管事一职，亚南因此能留于少林寺。

　　凡入寺者，不论僧俗及上下职位，一律强使习武每日全体同练武二时，亚南也不例外，某日亚南外出采办，经过丛林间，忽然听见雀鸟发出凄历之声，因而好奇，游目四望，果然在不远松树上，目睹一螳螂与相思雀对持突见该雀疾快向螳螂之头啄去随即见螳螂举双臂向其劈去，该雀惨叫一声，闪翼下堕于地，不能动弹，亚南惊奇疾向前发现其雀鸟颈处一线红丝，血渍斑斑。显然是螳螂之臂劈伤，亚南自小就天资聪明于是灵感一触，何不仿螳螂之法创出此拳。

　　此后亚南便捕捉一些螳螂回去，每日以草秆挑斗螳螂，观其格斗方法，因此也悟出一些套路拳法寺中无人知晓，有日亚南在□□□□螳螂拳法，恰逢禅隐大师经过，观其拳法并非少林拳种，大师高□□□□，责问亚南何来此拳法，亚南不敢隐瞒，便告诉禅隐大师此拳是从□□中所悟得来，禅隐大师惊奇称亚南是练武奇才，以加予指导大可造就，于是禅隐大师便将一些南少林拳法融入其中。

　　亚南加予苦练，终于成就，在国术中流一异彩的南派螳螂拳，不久亚南便南返广东东江一带开馆授徒，从学者皆为客家人居多，其中知名弟子黄福高宗师，经惠阳商贸时，来到惠阳古镇观音阁，将此拳传于刘水宗师。

Introduction of
East River Southern Praying Mantis Martial Arts

Introduction of
East River Southern Praying Mantis Martial Arts

Southern Praying Mantis Martial Art was founded in the Ching Dynasty. The founding father was a Shaolin cook, Chu Ah Nam (Chu Ya Nan) from Jiaying, Guangdong (now Guangdong, Xingning). Ah Nam belonged to a well to do peasant generation. He ended up with some kind of gastric illness and went about looking for a cure everywhere, but in vain. A friend of his father thought the disease could be caused by the local climate, water and soil and so advised him to travel around and seek for a prestigious herbal doctor to cure his stubborn disease. With no hope for his son's illness if he stayed home, Ah Nam's father agreed to this suggestion and financed Ah Nam and an old servant, Ah Yong, to set out and instructed Ah Nam to try to do business everywhere they went.

Finally, he said farewell to the family and travelled along Northern Guangdong, through Jiangxi, Hunan, and Fujian. Due to this exhausting long journey, servant Ah Yong was ill for months even with medical treatment, and ended up without hope and died. After the funeral of Ah Yong, Ah Nam later became very ill and most of his money was exhausted, so he tried to write home for help. But a slow remedy could not meet the urgency of the situation. Ah Nam despaired and was in deep worry. Fortunately the owner of a hostel, a kind man, old Yuan, knew Ah Nam was in such a helpless situation and offered him money and introduced him to a monk, Chan Yin, of the Southern Shaolin Temple, who was a prestigious medical expert and a master of Shaolin martial art. After receiving the monk's herbal medical treatment, Ah Nam recovered from his chronic stomach disease.

So far away from his home, Ah Nam worried about his day to day material living. Old Yuan, the hostel owner knew what was in Ah Nam's mind, and so asked Ah Nam whether he would like to have a job in the Shaolin Temple to make a living. "No matter how hard and tough the job, I am willing to take it" replied Ah Nam. Old Yuan told Master Chan Yin who pitied Ah Nam with sympathy and let Ah Nam manage the cooking section in the temple. And so, Ah Nam finally settled down in the Shaolin Temple.

No matter in high or low position in the Shaolin Temple, it was compulsory for everyone to practise two hours Kungfu training

Introduction Cont'd

everyday without fail. This was one of the rules of the temple. Ah Nam was no exception and had naught but to obey that.

One day, when Ah Nam was out to manage purchases, on the way through the woods, he suddenly heard some kind of crying painful sounds. Ah Nam curiously looked around and saw a praying mantis fighting with a red billed bird in a tree. The bird tried to peck the mantis head briskly, but the mantis was fending it off and attacked the bird with the sharp claws of its two arms. The mantis clawed at the neck of the bird which then fell on the ground with painful chirps...motionless the bird laid.

Ah Nam was surprised to notice there was a bloody cut on the neck of the bird. It apparently was cut was from the mantis. Well, Ah Nam was sharp and bright since his boyhood and all the sudden he comprehended an idea to imitate the mantis with his fists. Ah Nam then collected some mantids and irritated them with straws. Watching their movements he worked out a set of Praying Mantis martial arts which no one knew in the temple. And so this begot the name of Praying Mantis martial arts.

One day, Master Chan Yin passed by and saw Ah Nam practising Mantis martial arts and noticed this was not Shaolin kungfu. Delighted with cheer, he wanted to know where this art was from. Ah Nam revealed to the Master that he comprehended it from the praying mantis, and surprisingly, the Master proclaimed Ah Nam a genius in martial arts, and stated he could be outstanding in this field. Master Chan Yin also integrated his Shaolin Fist with Ah Nam's Praying Mantis martial arts thereafter.

With that, Ah Nam through the continuous endeavour of practising, made it to the highest level of Mantis Arts and flourished in his own right. Later Ah Nam came back to the East Guangdong area and established a Kungfu Institute teaching Mantis.

Most of the students are Hakka people and Master Wong Fook Go was one of them. While doing trades in Huiyang, Huizhou, Wong came to Guanyin Temple where he passed this Praying Mantis martial arts out to our Grandteacher Lao Sui, as a rare precious heritage. ###

东江三虎之——刘水（诚初）宗师履历

　　刘水宗师于1879年出生于广东省惠阳县芦岚香园围村刘屋，兄弟六个，自幼爱好武术，少年时期习有马家拳术，矮马功夫，还自创刘水棍棍术，二十岁时已拳棍非常了得。后在博罗观音阁遇到一个由广东兴宁在观音阁行医卖药叫黄福高的武术师，黄福高拳师看中刘水是一个习武的上料，故试比刘水功力，几个回合皆被黄师制服，刘水即下跪拜黄师为师，经过几年在黄师的教导下练就一身过硬的东江朱家螳螂拳棍跌打刀伤枪伤药等。学成后在二十多岁去香港发展，在香港红堪保其利街52号二楼开设武馆受徒学武，徒弟甚众，名徒如：朱冠华、朱植五、杨寿、谢松、谭华、林华、马森、邹文治、叶瑞等等。刘宗师为人耿直、豪爽、大义、以武德教育众徒，学武先学德，故所受众徒都是武德双全的优秀弟子，后在众徒之资助下，于1936年在老家香园围筑有祖屋一栋，当地人叫此屋"刘屋洋楼"，但遗憾的是当祖屋就要俊工时（即1941年冬）刘宗师想回家看看，恰遇日本鬼侵入中国香港伦陷，交通阻塞，而未能回家，后因思家心切，积虑于心，于1942年因病而度完了他人生64岁年华，故所以他一生劳碌积署造成的洋楼祖屋都没有亲身看上一眼。这不单是他个人的遗憾，也是众多亲人及众徒的遗憾。他的一生业绩只好留给他弟弟刘富元的后人留念及享用，而欣喜的是他的跌打刀伤、枪伤药法治疗传受给他的弟弟刘富元及其子孙代代相传，治疗百姓利民。

　　刘水宗师的螳螂拳后传有人，如：在香港武林界中承认的就有：杨寿、谢松、朱植伍、胡源、叶喜称为五虎将。还有朱观华、林华、谭华、谭照、孙兴、叶瑞、马铭森 在香港及英国、澳洲、西班牙、葡萄牙等国都发展为几千个弟子，在惠州后人也有陈建明、谢添胜、郭连相、刘论发、张仁全、罗煜明、薛观梅、马日良等几十个人，在中山有、林润字等几十个人。

Lao Sui (Liu Shui)
Grandmaster of Praying Mantis Martial Arts
One of the East River Three Tigers
Biography (following page)

Lao Sui
Grandmaster of Praying Mantis Martial Arts
One of the East River Three Tigers
Biography

Lao Sui was born in 1879, at Lunan, Xiang Yuan Village, Huiyang, Huizhou, Guangdong Province. He had six brothers and was fond of martial arts since his childhood. He practised Ma's fist boxing, a short horse kungfu. He himself created Lao's Pole styles and his own fist art ways. He excelled in the staff and fist martial arts by his 20s.

Later, he met a travelling herbal seller named Wong Fook Go in Boluo County, at Guanyin Temple. Wong, the medicine seller, noticed Lao Sui had good potential for a martial art career, and in order to try out Lao's kungfu level, challenged him to a fist fight. After a few rounds, Lao Sui was completely overwhelmed. So, he no sooner said than done, prostrated himself and knelt down in front of Wong, asking him to become a pupil.

After a few years from the teaching of Master Wong, Lao Sui became firm, strong, tough, and reached an outstanding level in Chu's Praying Mantis. In addition to the boxing, he trained staff, as well as herbal medicine for wounds and cuts, guns and knives and the likes thereof. After the completion of his training from Wong, Lao Sui went to Hong Kong to develop his career. He opened his martial art Institute on the 1st floor, at Polly Street, Hong Hum, in Kowloon and started taking students. There were quite a lot of prestigious disciples such as: Chu Kwong Wah, Chu Zhi Ng, Yang Shou, Tse Chun, Tan Wah, Lam Wah, Ma Sum, Chow Wen Chi, Ip Sui and others.

Grand master Lao Sui was straight forward, high minded, loyal, just, and wise. He instilled noble thoughts and morality in his students. Morality was the key approach and learning martial art was second. Thus, all his followers excelled in both morality and martial art.

In 1936, a building was contributed to master Lao Sui by his students in his home town of Xiang Yuan village. The people there called this building "Lao's Western House". Unfortunately, in 1941, during the completion of the house, Japanese invaders overran Hong Kong, and all transportations were blocked. And although, Grand Master Lao Sui desperately wanted to go home to see his house, his dream could not come true and he reached the end of his life, at the age of 64. He toiled his whole life and obtained this house, yet, in the end, he didn't even have a look at it with his own eyes. That was not only to his regret, but all his students, relatives and all the people who knew him. His heritage was then inherited by the generations of his brother Lao Fu Yuan. Until today, they still use herbal medicines, in this home, to cure wounds and treat folks and many people have benefitted from Lao Sui's heritage.

Grandmaster Liu Sui's Chu Family Praying Mantis martial arts passed to several generations too, with notables like Yang Sou, Tse Chong, Chu Zhi Ng, Fu Yuan, and Ip Hay. These five were named "Five Tiger Generals". Also, Chu Kwong Hua, Lam Wah, Tam Wah, Tam Jiu, Sun Hing, Yip Sui, and Ma Ming Sen were known as "Official Conductors" of Chu Gar Mantis.

In Hong Kong, Britain, Australia, Spain, and Portugal there are thousands of followers who train Lao Sui's legacy of Chu Gar Praying Mantis kungfu.

The descendants also in Huizhou, China are Chen Jian Ming, Tse Tim Sheng, Kwok Lian Shiun, Liu Lun Fa, Zhang Yuen Chuen, Lo Wong Ming, Si Kun May, Ma Yat Liang and others. In Zhongshan, China also there is Lin Yuen Yue who has taught many others. ###

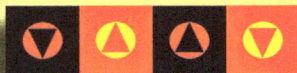

马铭森师义履历

　　马森（铭森）于1907年生于惠阳芦岚香园围塊籽祖屋，其父马贵清是刘水崇师的结拜同年兄弟，所以马森与刘水崇师是叔侄关系，马森欲呼刘为"同年爷"因其父亲马贵清早年长亲，二十岁时便去南洋新加坡谋生。

　　森于1934年27岁前去父亲处（新加坡）住宿2年，并于1936年在新加坡带回结发妻郑玉妹回香园老家安居，又在1937年去香港拜"同年爷"刘水学武五年，在五年学武时间里，非常刻苦，因刘崇师收徒甚众，森天天都要与几十年徒弟对练打绞槌，对双、单桩，提子，几乎天天如此，所以能练就一身过硬功夫，于1941年离港回香园围老家，以后再也无去过香港。回来老家30年时间从未表露过功夫，森为人忠厚，重武德，从不以武欺人，以品德善而择徒受之。

　　就在1972年，惠州陈建明当时十五岁，来香园拜森为师，当时社会气氛正不敢公开学武，又在1978年改革开放后，才开始从好朋友中教徒学习拳师者甚众，但真正学成者甚少，刘水崇师的朱豪东江螳螂拳拳种，在惠州水一带就只有马森一人传受此拳法，于1996年农历二月初三度过了他90岁的人生。

　　马森墓地于2003年12月建于寺园围南山下象壁山顶，墓名叫卧狮望江墓碑上刻上陈建明、谢澡胜、林润宇、罗煜明、卓述相、刘论发、张仁金、薛屺梅八位门生，以作后辈留念。此墓地得于其门徒林润宇在中山著名风水师，找遍千山山脉才得此地。其徒林润宇对师傅之情从此墓地可表其心也。

Ma Ming Sen Biography
Son-in-law of Lao Sui

Ma Sen (Ming Sen) was born 1907. His native home is Lunan, Xiang Yuan Village, Huiyang, Huizhou, Guangdong Province. His father, Ma Gui Qing, was a sworn brother and the same age as Lao Sui. Ma Ming Sen called Lao Sui "Grandpa" - although he was the same age as his own father but they were Uncle and Nephew in relationship as Lao Sui and his father were sworn brothers. Because Ma Ming Sen's mother died early, his father Ma Gui Qing then went abroad to South East Asia and Singapore to make his living. He was in his 20s.

When Ma Ming Sen was 27, (1934), he joined his father in Singapore and lived there for two years. In 1936, he returned to his native home in Huiyang and settled down with his wife Cheng Yuk Mei, who he married in Singapore. By 1937, he went to Hong Kong to visit Grandmaster Lao Sui and learned martial art from him for some five years. During that period of time, Ma Ming Sen worked extremely hard in practising Kungfu martial arts with Master Lao Sui's tens of disciples everyday without fail. He trained all the sets of movements, face to face attacks and defences. Thus, at his peak, he was strong, firm and tough, being in full possession of his Master Lao Sui's Chu Gar Praying Mantis.

In 1941, Ma Ming Sen left Hong Kong and went back to his native home and never returned to Hong Kong. For 30 years in his native home, he never demonstrated his kungfu openly to a soul. He was straightforward and honest, taking moral obligation as his first priority. He never bullied others and was very choosy in taking followers. Character, conduct and moral concepts were key requirements to enter the martial art door of Ma Ming Sen.

In 1972, when Chen Jian Ming was just 15 years old, he came from from Huizhou to Xiang Yuan village to prostrate himself before Ma Ming Sen as a pupil. However, in those years, learning or lecturing on martial arts was prohibited and no one dared cross this red line. Not until the opening up and reform of the country, did Ma take pupils from some acquaintances and friends. After all, only a handful of them were able to master the martial arts, anyway. Of all Grandmaster Lao Sui's Praying Mantis Kungfu seeds, Ma Ming Sen was the sole one to pass and spread the art back in the Huizhou hometown area.

In the 1996 Lunar Year of February 3rd, Ma Ming Sen passed away at the age of 90. Ma's tomb was built in February 2003 in his Xiang Yuan village, on the south peak of a hill overlooking the East River. The name of the tomb is "Lying Lion Viewing over the River". Eight disciple's names were inscribed on it as a memorial for coming generations. This tomb site was located and selected by a famous horoscope diviner from Zhongsan. The disciple Lin Lunyi made these efforts and it showed the deep devotion of Lin to Master Ma Ming Sen. The names of the 8 disciples were : Chen Jian Ming, Xie Tiansheng, Lin Lunyi, Lo Xue Ming, Guo Lianxiang, Liu Luan Fa, Zhang Ruanquan, and Xue Guanmei. ###

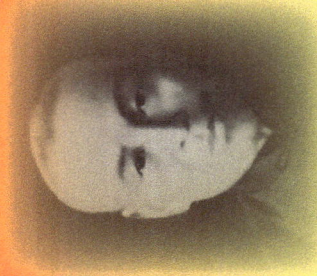

POETRY OF LAO SUI

Drift about from place to place
just for a living
Time slips by without achieving anything
Want to go home but not content with cloistered life
Familial affection is gone with the wind
Nowhere to find a pure land in the world
My motherland is now igniting into war
I have seen through the world of mortals clearly
I feel so desperate and all the hope turns to dust
Life to me is just like a dream

亲水人亲未新能与家谁多年生死嗟殊兄有团抚悠物千灭香作者

注：此诗是刘水宗师晚年思念亲人、思乡、感叹而作。

156

POETRY OF LAO SUI

Decades are wasted with nothing achieved
Spring flowers are blooming early in the
land of my sojourn

My heart is torn with anxiety about my hometown.
My hometown is closed off to all traffic due to war

I am willing to risk my life and slip into inland
My family ties are severed by the scourge of war

I am alone in a strange island

I feel powerless and could be only walled off in my
own worries

注：此诗是刘水宗师亲笔之作，因此

157

Note on Hand Names and Translations
In China, everyone has their own "jia xiang hua", or home town dialect. Hakka is one such dialect and each clan or town may even have their own pronunciation of Hakka language. The names given herein, are the names that are commonly used so that everyone is on the same page and understands which skill or hand is being talked about. It is less important what you call the skills, and more important that everyone understands.

The Chinese romanization herein is the same — it is written phonetically or what is common, so that it can be easily understood. Chinese names herein are not correct pinyin, purposely. All errors in the Chinese text are mine and not to be attributed to the editors.

"Shu, Sao, and Shou" all simply mean "hand" and are often used interchangeably. Remember, once the stance, root and feeling hand is skilled, the whole body is one "hand".

About Southern Mantis on the Internet
The internet and DVDs can be a great aid to learning. How much better are DVDs than secretly peeking through holes in a fence or wall to learn Mantis? In the early days, sneaking a peek through a hole was quite common.

Nothing can replace the spirit and hand of a skillful teacher. But, the new media and resources are still a valuable asset. The internet, however, is also a large source of disinformation. Repeating what someone else said erroneously often becomes accepted as SPM "truth" without verification. There is a great deal of "false" information on the internet about Southern Praying Mantis.

An example is the 'Blanco' article. Circa mid 1990s, Blanco, from Hong Kong, called my office in the USA asking how to contact Southern Mantis teachers in China. I did not provide him any information. Southern Mantis teachers usually frown on unannounced visits from strangers. Later, he "compiled" his article using sources, such as my published works, without permission. Much of his article is erroneous and needs correction. I encourage you to seek the truth for yourself. Do not follow any one blindly. Search and prove all things. The further you go downstream the murkier the water. Drink close to the source.

Errata:
Sifu Ma Jiuhua would like to state clearly that he was misquoted in the Dongjiang Times newspaper. He did not say that Chow Gar did not exist in China and he was misquoted by the reporter. He encourages everyone to come to China and search for themselves. What he said to the reporter was that the legacy of Lao Sui in China is and has always been Chu Gar Mantis from Chu Ya Nan in Wuhua, not Chow Gar. (Refer to my first book, Chu Gar Gao, for more information on the late Sifu Yip Sui and Chow Gar.)

Additional photos indicated ©今日惠州网，天鹅城网

Chu Gar Mantis Today
Many of Lao Sui's relatives train Chu Gar in China today. As stated earlier the Lao and Ma families have been neighbors for more than 100 years and their families have long been related by marriage. The Lao family and Ma families still live side by side in the old village area and both families carry Chu Gar Mantis forward and their ages range from teens to 95 years old. Among the Lao family who train are: Lao Xiang Nan, Lao Yue Gong, Lao Su Shen, Lao Zhen Zhong and Lao Wei Long. Among the Ma family are: Ma Jiuhua, Ma Wei Dong, Ma Yi Liang, Ma Wei Bo, Ma Wei Chao, Ma Wei Liang, Ma Jiu Hui, Ma Wei Ting, Ma Wei Zhen, Ma Wei Cho and others such as Guo Linxiang, Luo Xianming, Zhang Renquan, and Zhen Zihui, etc.

There are three Clans of Chu Gar teaching and all are descended from Ma Mingsen. Sifu Chen Jianming teaches in Huicheng. Sifu Xie Tiansheng in Boluo and Sifu Lin Lunyi in Zhongsan. This is in addition to those who train and teach privately.

Miscellanies

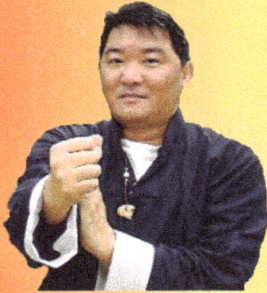

Special thanks to Dr. Simon Han, Taiwan Cardiologist and Weng Chun Boxing teacher, for his time spent editing the Chinese text in this book. You may contact Dr. Han directly by email to discuss Taiwan martial art and for Hakka Mantis training in Taipei, Taiwan - simonclh@gmail.com.

Also, Uncle Cheung Ting and Ms. Huang Yan for their valuable contributions to the Chinese text and this book.

雜記

手法名稱和翻譯

在中國人人有自己的家鄉話或方言。客家話也是一種方言，雖然同屬客家人，但因地理隔閡，客家話的發音及表達用詞常有明顯的出入，

因此我們對每丨手法的名稱和譯名著重於溝通，而非精準而統一的命名，英文音譯名遵循原始方言的發音，但非今日標準漢語拼音，如"shu、 sao，shou"都只是"手"的音譯，經常交互使用。

＊請記住純熟穩固的樁馬和手法將整個身體整合為手。

南方螳螂在互聯網

互聯網和教學光碟對於學習大有助益。但透過教學光碟會比通過柵欄或牆縫偷學更好嗎？在早期偷學是很常見的事。

事實上沒有任何媒體可以取代老師的精神和純熟的手法。但是不可否認的，媒體和網路資源對學習仍然是相當有助益。然而互聯網也是錯誤知識的最大源頭，常見的錯誤就是未經查證而無條件接受別人錯誤的見解，事實上在互聯網上就存在大量的南方螳螂虛假資訊。

大約在 90 年代中期，有人從香港聯繫我，希望我提供中國南方螳螂拳老師的聯絡訊息以便撰寫專文，我沒有提供他任何資訊，因為我知道南方螳螂拳老師通常不喜歡被陌生人打擾，後來

他依循我發表的文章編寫了他自己的文章，可想而知他的文章是錯誤百出，我鼓勵所有對南方螳螂拳有興趣的人自己尋求真理，不要盲從，搜尋並查證所有的資料，應溯溪而上尋找源頭。

勘誤：

馬九華師傅清楚地聲明東江時報的記者對他的訪談有些出入，他鼓勵大家自行來中國查證，他對記者說： 劉水在中國的所傳源自於五華朱亞南的朱家螳螂拳。（參閱我第一本書"朱家螳螂拳"後段葉瑞師傅與周家螳螂拳）。

附加照片 © 今日惠州網，天鵝城網

今日朱家螳螂拳在廣東

很多劉水在中國的後人仍學習家傳的朱家螳螂拳，如前文所述的劉水和馬銘森家族比鄰而居且聯姻已經超過百年，他們家族仍居住於劉水故鄉，從十幾歲到九十五歲老人仍然積極練習朱家螳螂拳。他們包括： 劉湘南，劉瑞光，劉 Sushen，劉振忠，劉威龍；馬家族人有：馬九華，馬偉東，馬日梁，馬偉波，馬偉橋，馬九良，馬九輝，馬偉庭，馬偉軍，馬偉珠，其他為： 郭連相，羅煜明，張仁全，曾志輝，林潤宇等等。

馬銘森傳人公開教學者則有惠城區陳建明師傅，博羅的謝添勝師傅和中山的 林潤宇 師傅。 還有其他的一些人。

特別感謝韓志陸博士
（澳大利亞國立昆士蘭大學血管生物學哲學博士）
韓志陸博士為臺北榮民總醫院成人心臟科主治醫師和永春拳教師，他耗費許多時間翻譯校對本書中文，您可以直接透過電子郵件（simonclh@gmail.com）與他聯絡，討論武術和客家螳螂拳的訓練。

此外， 還感謝叔叔張庭和女士黃艷為本書的貢獻。

161

A Final Note

The present is the living sum-total of the whole past. While they still exist, we have the benefit of questioning, hand to hand and face to face, the elders regarding Southern Mantis history and original transmission. However, the elders with first hand knowledge and experience, are less and less with every day passing. Only a handful remain.

This book relates to the basic history of Chu Gar Mantis and Lao Sui's legacy in China. My first Volume, *Chu Gar Gao*, addressed Lao Siu's Chu Gar legacy in Hong Kong.

The three branches of Southern Praying Mantis are from one root. Each has its advantage and is worthy of study. Although, I am first, Kwongsai Jook Lum Temple Mantis, and second, Chu Gar Mantis, both by Ceremony and Transmission, I am not biased or preferential. They are harmonious and may be taught side by side. The only difference is the depth of the transmission one receives.

Train Southern Mantis by DVD or come to Hong Kong and China to study Southern Mantis. Join my class. Email me directly. Welcome!

最后需要注意

目前就是活生生的整个过去的总和。虽然他们仍然存在着，我们有质疑的效益，手手和面对面，关于南部螳螂历史和原始的传输的长老。然而的长老与第一手知识和经验，，越来越少的每一天的传递。只有极少数保持。
这本书涉及到朱家螳螂和刘水遗留在中国的历史。我的第一卷，朱家教，解决刘水朱家遗留在香港。
三个分支的南部螳螂是从一个根。每个有它的优势，是值得研究。虽然我是第一，江西竹林寺螳螂，，第二，朱家螳螂，既由仪式和传输，我没有偏见或优待。他们是和睦的也可以教他们一起。唯一的区别是一个接收的传输的深度。
你想学 DVD 还是来到中国，学南部螳螂，然后你可以直接电子邮件通知我。加入我的课。欢迎您 们！

Roger D. Hagood
Standing Chairman
rdh@chugarmantis.com
www.chugarmantis.com

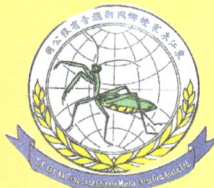

Hong Kong Chu Gar Tonglong Martial Art Association Headquarters

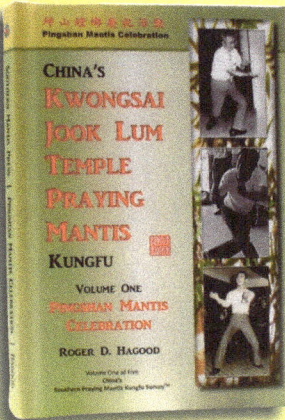
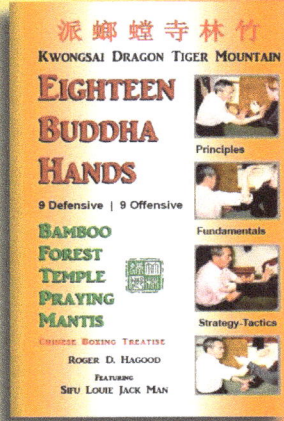
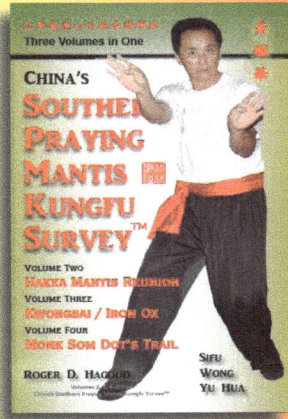
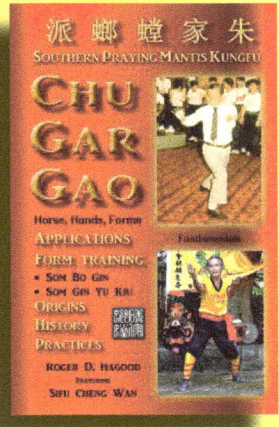
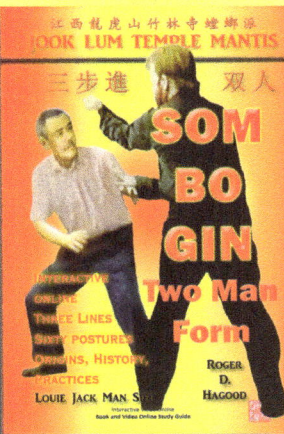
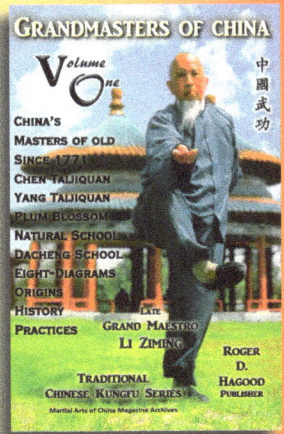

ChinaMantis.com   Instructional DVDs

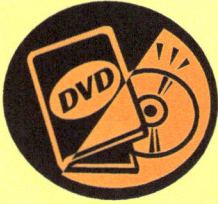

Jook Lum Temple Mantis Step by Step Instruction in 18 Volumes

Year One Training
Volume One: Fundamentals; The Most Important
Volume Two: Phoenix Eye Fist Attacking / Stepping
Volume Three: Centerline Defense
Volume Four: One, Three & Nine Step Attack / Defense
Volume Five: Centerline Sticky Hand Training
Volume Six: Same Hand / Opposite Hand Attacks
Volume Seven: Sai Shu, Sik Shu, Jik (Chun) Shu
Volume Eight: Gow Choy; Hammer Fist-Internal Strength
Volume Nine: Footwork in Southern Praying Mantis
Volume 10:   Chi Sao Sticky Hands and Passoffs

Advanced Two Man Forms — Year Two and Three
Available by request. Prerequisite Volumes 1– 10.
Volume 11: Loose Hands One
Volume 12: Som Bo Gin
Volume 13: Second Loose Hands
Volume 14: 108 Subset
Volume 15: Um Hon One
Volume 16: Um Hon Two
Volume 17: Mui Fa Plum Flower
Volume 18: Eighteen Buddha Hands
All 8 two man forms must be trained as one continuous set on both A - B sides.

DVD Descriptions and Video Clips
http://www.southernmantispress.com/southern-praying-mantis-instructional-dvds.htm

Summary Year One
http://www.chinamantis.com/first-year-training.htm

香港朱家螳螂鄭運國術體育會

HK CHU KA TONG LONG CHENG WAN MARTIAL ART ASSOCIATION

聘任證書　證字第壹佰零捌號

茲敦聘

ROGER D. HAGOOD

為本會

第廿九屆名譽會長

此聘

香港朱家螳螂鄭運國術體育會

香港總會會長：馬國宏
總會長：朱上星冠雄
會長：朱國威
長：朱修國威勤

主席：夏朱國威
名譽主席：黃朱國偉
主任：朱管國國
術副主任：鄭夏管國
術副主任：朱管國國

RDH Appointed Standing Chairman in 2002

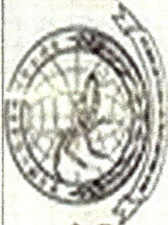

二〇〇二年　六月　九日

Study Mantis in China with the Author!

Your email correspondence is welcome and do visit and study Hakka Southern Praying Mantis with me in beautiful sunny south China! I am an Author, Publisher and Producer of eBooks, books, journals, videos and 7 International martial arts newsstand magazines in 15 countries with 45 years in training and teaching martial arts and some 20 years living in China and Asia!

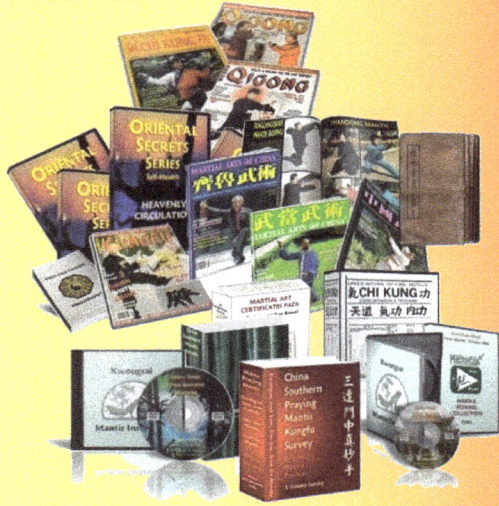

Currently residing in beautiful sunny south China for the last 10 years where I teach Southern Praying Mantis. Join my class in Guangdong today!

您的電子郵件通信是受歡迎的過來上我的課我教你客家螳螂在美麗陽光南中國！

作者+客家螳螂師傅、 出版商和生產商的電子圖書、 書籍、 期刊、 錄影和 7個 國際武術書報攤雜雜誌在 15 個國家中有 45 年的培訓和教學武術和一些生活在中國和亞洲的 20 年！

目前居住在美麗的陽光南中國那裡我教南螳螂在過去 10 年。今天歡迎你們加入我在廣東省的課！

RDH, Pingshan Town, Guangdong, China, Summer, 2013
中國廣東省深圳市坪山鎮2013年夏

More Bio:
http://www.chugarmantis.com/publisher-s-page-2.htm
http://www.chinamantis.com/roger-d.-hagood.htm
Email: rdh@chinamantis.com

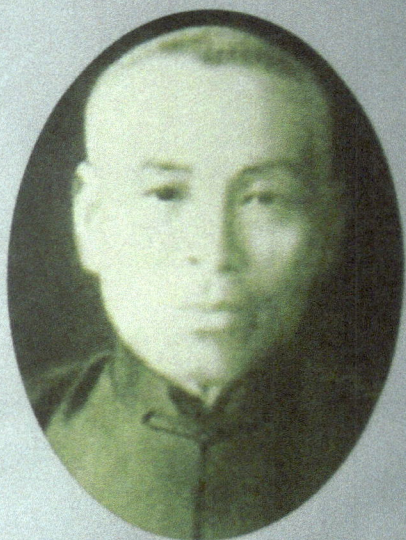

Lao Sui - 3rd Generation Chu Gar Gao

像遺公師水劉

螳螂江東

學仁學儀學功夫

遵親遵師遵教訓

像遺公初誠號水劉
(1879-1942)

Huiyang, Huizhou

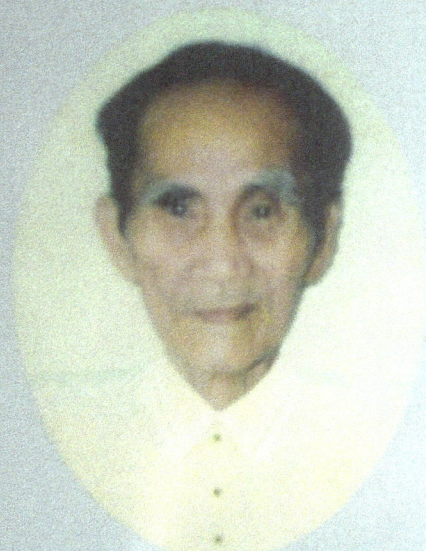

Ma Mingsen - 4th Generation Chu Gar Gao

像遺公師森銘马

東江螳螂

正直做人

學武強身

銘森公遺像

(1907-1996)

Guangdong, China

www.ingramcontent.com/pod-product-compliance
Lightning Source LLC
Chambersburg PA
CBHW040406110426
42812CB00011B/2472